RESEARCHING AIDS, SEXUALITY AND GENDER

Zapf Chancery Policy on Peer-Reviewing

All scholarly and academic works published by Zapf Chancery are peer-reviewed by at least two scholars in the field to which the work belongs. The purpose of peer reviewing is to get a second opinion from the community of scholarship to which the author belongs and thus add value to the work. All peer-reviewing is "blind-reviewing," that is, the reviewer does not get to know the author, nor does the author get to know the reviewer.

Peer-reviewing is done with the help of a specially designed instrument awarding numerical score on originality (40%), quality and currency of the sources cited (20%), presentation (30%), and language & Style (10%). For a work to be published a minimum cumulative score of 60 per cent on the British grading scale is required. Works falling below this score are referred back to authors for improvement and further reviewing until the desired score can be obtained.

****

Zapf Chancery Peer Reviewers (among others subject specific)

Prof. Joseph Galgalo, PhD (Cantab.), Vice Chancellor and Associate Professor of Theology, St. Paul's University, Limuru, Kenya; Prof. Esther Mombo, PhD, DD (HC), Deputy Vice Chancellor (Academics) and Associate Professor of Church History and Gender Theology, St. Paul's University, Limuru, Kenya; Rev. CB Peter, PhD (Cand), Senior Lecturer in Biblical Studies and Theology, St. Paul's University, Limuru, Kenya; Prof. Chris L. Wanjala, Professor of Literature, University of Nairobi, Kenya; Dr. Godwin Siundu, PhD, Senior Lecturer in English and Literature, University of Nairobi, Kenya; Mr. Enoch Harun Opuka, BEd, MPhil, Development Education Pratitioner; Dr John Blevins, ThD, Associate Professor of Research, Rollins School of Public Health, Emory University, Atlanta Georgia, USA; Prof. M. J. Kelly, Zambia

Researching AIDS, Sexuality and Gender

Case Studies of Women in Kenyan Universities

SECOND REVISED EDITION

Prof. Nyokabi Kamau MA, MPhil, PhD

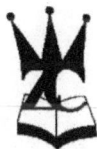

Zapf Chancery
Limuru, Kenya

First published 2009
Revised edition 2013

Copyright © Nyokabi Kamau 2013

Cover concept and design
Ediprint Communications

Design and typesetting
Ediprint Communications
P.O. Box 1207-00902, Kikuyu
Email: ediprint@yahoo.co.uk

Set in Book Antiqua 11 on 13.5

Printed in Kenya by
Kijabe Printing Press
P.O. Box 40
Kijabe

Published by

Zapf Chancery Publishers Africa Ltd.
c/o St. Paul's University,
P.O. Private Bag,
Limuru - 00217, Kenya.
Email: info@zapfchancery.org
Website: www.zapfchancery.org
Mobile: 0721-222-311

ISBN: 978-9966-040-29-9

To my late grandmother, Nyokabi wa Waiganjo,
for all her love and strong belief in my abilities
ever since I was a small girl.
May she rest in eternal peace.

Contents

Foreword

AIDS and People

The real, unspeakable tragedy of the AIDS epidemic is the destruction of people through the infection, illness or death of individuals. We must never overlook all that is going on at this individual, personal level. Behind all the mind-boggling AIDS statistics are men, women and children, experiencing a heartbreaking mixture of fear and anxiety, bodily pain and physical disability, isolation and rejection, loneliness and depression, anger and guilt, stigma and self-accusation. No matter how much we see on television or read in newspapers about HIV or AIDS, we must never forget the individual human beings who are affected. It is their personal situation that we want to remedy. It is their tragic situation that impels us to do what we can to understand the epidemic, reduce its transmission, and lessen its numerous impacts.

The evidence of this very powerful book is that senior highly educated women academics experience these impacts just as other people do. Their educational accomplishments and their generally high social status do not protect them. Indeed, if anything, they aggravate the situation for them. They suffer greatly from the epidemic. They experience its many negative effects. They feel powerless in relation to it. They are at a loss as to where they should turn, given the silence and effective denials within which the epidemic continues to be enshrouded, in university circles as much as (if not more than) elsewhere.

Women and AIDS in Universities

Throughout this book, Prof. Kamau presents us with what senior university women have to say on the double tragedy that HIV and AIDS represent in their lives: the failure of their institutions to give them (and no doubt countless others who are equally affected) the support they need in their AIDS-affected condition, and the way their status as women worsens every aspect of this condition. From the evidence presented it is clear that in the universities investigated there was an almost complete lack of initiatives to deal with HIV and AIDS, especially in their effects on women. There were few signs of institutionalised responses to the epidemic, not to mention the responses that took account of the different ways the epidemic affects women and men.

That this study represents the position as late as 2004–2005, the years of the investigation, demonstrates that universities have failed to internalise and act upon two messages: that there is a compelling case for every university to respond in a coherent and institutionalised manner to the AIDS epidemic; and, that there is an equally compelling case for every university to show delicate gender sensitivity in all its operations, especially in matters relating to senior women staff.

Universities Responding to HIV and AIDS

It is with an unhappy sense of déjà vu that one reads Prof. Kamau's words; that in the area of HIV and AIDS, universities were almost exclusively concerned with the welfare of students, but showed much less concern about the welfare of their academic staff. Recurring themes in evaluations of university responses to the epidemic have been that academic institutions know little about how HIV is affecting them; that students feature more strongly than staff at the centre of whatever little activity there may be; that institutionalising an HIV response appears as something quite new, poorly understood, and not happening in an effective sustainable way; and, that HIV and AIDS initiatives are mostly sporadic, uncoordinated and dependent on the initiatives of a few dedicated staff and students. It is unfortunate that it continues to be so in the universities that were investigated and that so little is being done to galvanise a vigorous and proactive response to the epidemic.

What HIV and AIDS Do

Looked at analytically, HIV and AIDS can be said to do three things:

1. They highlight and call for reform in existing problem areas, such as the absence of workplace structures for dealing with personal issues, the lack of gender equity, the existence of gender-based violence, or the existence of discriminatory power structures.

2. They magnify the scale and complexity of ongoing problems, such as achieving the third Millennium Development Goal of reducing global poverty and hunger in a world where HIV and AIDS undermine food security, or ensuring that programmes for infrastructural development take full account of HIV implications and vulnerabilities.

3. They create new problems, such as ensuring that in high prevalence countries every university graduate is equipped with the competence to deal with the disease and its impacts, personally in their own lives and professionally in their area of expertise, or developing the teaching materials that will make it possible for primary and secondary school teachers to incorporate HIV and AIDS into their teaching work

In her work, Prof. Kamau brings out the reality of this triple impact within the universities that she investigated. Within these institutions she finds that HIV and AIDS are inexorably leading to a greater awareness of existing problems, enlarged and more complex ongoing problems, and fresh challenges, especially for women.

Patriarchy is Ever-Present

The perspective of how senior women academics have been affected by the epidemic leads quickly to an examination of the way workplaces in universities are still governed by deeply rooted patriarchal power structures and practices that express the strong entrenchment of male superiority and domination over women.

The recognition of these inequitable power structures leads almost automatically to the challenge to university systems to move away from patriarchal structures and towards the provision of equal opportunities for all employees.

The book makes a strong case that women should never feel silenced when bringing their personal experiences into the workplace or the public domain because what they experience in their private and personal capacity as women who manage households, or are wives and mothers, has ramifications for their opportunities and accomplishments in the public sphere. Their very experience of HIV within themselves, their families or communities accentuates how deeply they realise that for them "the personal is political".

Stigma, Sexuality and HIV

In 1987, in an address to the United Nations General Assembly, Jonathan Mann, founder of the Global Programme on AIDS, UNAIDS predecessor, noted that in HIV and AIDS we are confronted not with one, but with three epidemics. First, there is the developmental epidemic of HIV. This strikes silently and can go undetected for ten years or more. But throughout the course of those years it does two things: it steadily undermines and destroys the body's defence mechanisms, and it makes the person in whom it resides infectious, capable of passing the virus on to others. Second, there is the medical epidemic of visible AIDS or AIDS-related illnesses, with all their debilitating and life-threatening manifestations. Third, there is the social epidemic of the stigma and discrimination that grinds people down in shame, isolation and rejection.

The findings of Prof. Kamau's study show that attitudes of denial and AIDS-related stigma continue to plague African universities. This was expressly acknowledged by the Director of the AIDS Control Unit at one of the institutions investigated: "Our biggest challenge is stigma amongst our staff members. There are still very many who cannot come and tell us what their problems are." A major reason for this stigma is one that invariably appears in the literature on AIDS-related stigma, the tendency to moralise the issue and make a false identification between HIV and sin, to blame AIDS on sin. As Prof. Kamau points out, "The linking of AIDS to promiscuity in women seems to cause stigma and silence, especially amongst educated and Christian women who would not want to be associated with such a disease."

The paralysing anguish and shame of all forms of stigma owe much to this human propensity to associate HIV infection with moral failure. Seemingly in some radical way we humans are not able to cope with the notion that sexual activity, which should be the channel of ecstatic joy and the possibility of new life, should instead be the route to destructive and dehumanising illnesses and possible death. This concern that a fundamental purpose of our sexuality has gone seriously wrong seems to be so deeply rooted in our human psyche that we make use of a moral framework to talk about it and set the parameters within which it can surface. But this harmful identification between HIV infection and moral failure must be fought tooth and nail. Educators, university leaders, public persons, religious leaders, and all others need to be fearless and tireless in persuading people to accept the message: HIV is not a sin. AIDS is not a sin. The real sin, if the term must be used, is stigma and individuals and communities must spare no efforts in rooting this out.

Integral to this approach is the need to help people develop a more positive attitude to sex and sexuality, as Prof. Kamau repeatedly stresses. There is need for every leader, especially for religious leaders, to proclaim the inherent goodness of the human body and all those feelings, moods and emotions that bring two people together in a creative intimacy of closeness and love. Every advance in this direction will help in dismantling the association between HIV and conduct that is labelled as immoral. By the same token, it will help in neutralising the way moralising attitudes buttress stigma and discrimination.

The Silences that Must be Overcome

In a brilliant summary Prof. Kamau outlines how a combination of feminist and HIV perspectives makes it possible to see the unseen, name the unnamed and unearth silences that exist in different areas of women's lives and in the universities. Guided by the powerful words of Hilary Clinton, "too many women, in too many countries, speak the same language of silence", the investigation finds that educated and well-off women have been silenced by the current debates about HIV and AIDS in Africa, which have continued to focus on behaviour models. In the AIDS and university context, silence refers to those issues, especially those concerning women, that are unspoken, taken for granted, or seen as though they cannot be challenged. Such issues are ignored because it is believed that this is the way they should be – mainly because they favour men – in a patriarchal system that characterises the functioning of society not just in Kenya, but also in almost every other part of the world.

Breaking these silences remains a major task for society and its institutions, including universities:

- Silence about what is known but not taken into account, as with universities' choice to remain silent about the impacts of AIDS on their staff, although they are aware of its devastating effects.

- Silence about issues that people may feel constrained to talk about, such as the inability of educated women to talk about HIV and AIDS in relation to their own experience, largely because of the taboos surrounding the discourse about sex.

- Silence about not knowing issues, with professional women seeing no unfairness in the way society positions them, being unwilling to challenge the status quo, and accepting as a non-negotiable principle that they should do everything in their power to support their husbands and families while still trying their best to manage their careers.

- Silence about issues that are seen to belong to the private sphere, with women experiencing powerlessness to bring into the workplace, where the dominant culture is that of male hegemony, control and supremacy, matters from the private sphere that greatly affect their performance as academics, university employees and managers of households.

- Silence and fear induced by views that HIV and AIDS come from morally reprehensible conduct and by the absence of suitable forums that would allow educated women to discuss sexuality and bring it out into the open.

- Silence about HIV infection that blocks senior women academics from presenting themselves for an HIV test.

- Silence about women's sexuality, the failure to discuss heterosexuality (especially within marriage), the bland hope that husbands would remain faithful or would use condoms whenever they chose to have sex outside marriage, and the stigma and silence surrounding lesbianism.

Conclusion: Breaking the Dominance of Patriarchy

One of the main findings of this study is that patriarchy dominates the AIDS discourse, not just in universities, but throughout Kenya and the world. This finding gives the book relevance beyond Kenya and the university world. But it is also very sobering, since few of the global, in-country or local responses to the epidemic incorporate any real attempt to address the issue of patriarchy. It seems to be something that is taken for granted and cannot be challenged in AIDS programmes. Yet, this may well be the elephant in the room that has largely been ignored at the great human cost of global failure to roll back the epidemic.

Prof. Kamau's book is a vibrant call for the dismantling of the entire dominant patriarchal structure. For more than sixty years the international community has given voice to the principle that can lead to such dismantling, Article 1 of the Universal Declaration of Human Rights: "All human beings are born free and equal in dignity and rights". What is needed is to turn these words into action.

This book proclaims the need for such action in universities and makes us aware of a similar need in all walks of life, because, notwithstanding its title, the book is not just about AIDS, sexuality and gender. It is about the most enduring, universal, comprehensive, wide-ranging injustice in the world – treating half the human race as if they were of lesser moment, denying them accomplishment, fulfilment and satisfaction if they do not conform to the conventions, dictates and cultures of male-dominated societies, ignoring the centrality of women's attitudes, values and concerns.

This is not the first book that has raised these issues, however, it is the first to raise them in the context of a world with AIDS and of universities that seem indifferent to their responsibility in such a world. How many more careful investigations do we need before we do something about this? How many more women must expend their energy as Prof. Kamau has done before the world wakes up to the flagrant way it is violating the free and equal dignity and rights of women, and thereby of men? When will we ever learn? When will we act? What are we waiting for? Surely this is the kairos moment, the time for deep recognition followed by decisive and transforming action.

In the world of AIDS, we are accustomed to hearing that it can no longer be business as usual. Prof. Kamau's insightful examination of one aspect of this world of AIDS provides powerful arguments for the even more basic affirmation that in the world of patriarchy it can no longer be business as usual. It would be a wonderful vindication of this book if every one of its readers would take this message right into their hearts and then go and do something about it.

Michael J. Kelly,
Lusaka, Zambia
2nd March, 2009

═Preface to the Second Revised Edition═

It has been eight years since this research was carried out and six years since the first edition of this book was issued. The first edition, which was published under the title AIDS, Sexuality and Gender: Experiences of Women in Kenyan Universities (2009), has been read widely by many graduate students and colleagues working in the area of HIV and AIDS around the world. There have been many encouraging comments on the book, particularly to the effect that it continues to address issues that are still relevant. The comments and encouragement received prompted me to fill the gaps in the first edition, especially in the area of researching a sensitive topic using a feminist methodology. This has been the main reason for working on this revised edition.

The findings of the research presented in this book formed the beginning of a more informed engagement with issues of gender, religion and sexuality. In this revised edition, not only have errors been corrected, but data and the reference list have also been updated. The tools used in the research have been included and placed in the Appendices section and the edition now carries an index. All this has been done to enhance the aspect of research in the publication.

After completing my doctoral studies, I was appointed a Director of the St Paul's Institute of Life Long Learning at St Paul's University, Kenya. This was a unique and challenging opportunity for me as I was also to be the coordinator of an international Masters programme on Community Pastoral Care and HIV and AIDS. This was the only HIV and AIDS Masters programme in the whole of Eastern Africa. It was being offered in collaboration with University of Wales, Lampeter.

One of my briefs upon employment was to revise the curriculum and present it to the Commission for Higher Education (CHE) so that St Paul's University could run it independently. The biggest challenge that my colleagues and I faced was to convince CHE that there was still need for an MA focusing on HIV and AIDS. They argued that this pandemic was now under control, and hence there was no need for such a programme. This was despite the fact that the HIV prevalence rate in Kenya was still above 6 per cent and there were still more than 2.5 million people living with the virus. Moreover, the challenges of stigma still remain. It was therefore a battle to convince the CHE committee that such a programme was still relevant in the 21st century.

We finally succeeded to convince the Commission, though with a much watered down curriculum. Much of the community aspect of the programme, which was to make it even more relevant, was removed. This aspect was to be relevant not just to the students, but also to the communities where the students served. This in itself was an indication of the silences around this pandemic that this study unearthed.

Of interest however, was that just like the two universities that were selected as the case studies in this book, I found that even at St Paul's University, there was hardly any specific activities that were directed at supporting members of staff especially those who may have been affected and/or infected by HIV and AIDS. Although by the year 2007 when I joined the university the situation had improved greatly with regard to access to treatment, there was no personal support for staff members. This was regardless of the fact that HIV and AIDS training had been fully mainstreamed in all the courses within the university.

St Paul's University was granted a full charter in October 2007, just a month after I joined. Before then, it had been a United Theological College whose main mandate was the training of pastors. Just like Holy Ghost University, St Paul's was also quite patriarchal and issues of women were hardly given priority. Some personal stories from the women who had been there for long showed that the issues that had emerged in the research presented in the book were still alive and well almost five years later. This was so even in a university that would have been considered to have done a lot with regard to HIV and AIDS; for instance, the university had an AIDS policy and a VCT on campus, but these were regarded as students' facilities rather than for members of staff.

It did not take me long to realise that the women members of staff had many personal issues to deal with, just like the women in the universities presented in this book. Luckily, at St Paul's, soon after the charter was awarded, a woman was appointed Deputy Vice Chancellor, Academics. This woman is a strong feminist theologian and she was well aware of the unique challenges that women face in universities, especially those with a predominantly masculine culture. She therefore shared with me the idea of a university women's fellowship that would bring together all the women members of staff to a safe place where they could provide support to one another on personal and professional issues.

In early 2008, this fellowship was formed and I became its first chair. As the chair, I had the privilege of putting to action some of the recommendations given in this book, especially that women need a space in the academy where their personal issues can also be seen to be political. To cut a long story short, this fellowship has grown to a strong movement of women of St Paul's where we celebrate each others' personal and professional achievements, comfort each other during hard times, and encourage each other to move to even greater heights within the institution and elsewhere. Even though issues of HIV and AIDS have not formed a prominent part of the fellowship's agenda, it has reached a point where we can now start inviting speakers to address the sensitive subject of sex and sexuality. The fellowship has also sponsored an orphan girl from a children's home located near the university to secondary school. It has promised to take care of her studies and other needs until she reaches university level after which another girl will be sponsored.

At the students' level, I was also keen to see the subject of sex and sexuality demystified and de-stigmatised. As a head of a newly formed Department of Arts and Social Sciences, I developed a common course on gender, sexuality and HIV and AIDS, which is taken by all undergraduate students who enrol at St Paul's University, regardless of the degree they are pursuing. At a personal level, I have continued to engage the best way I can with issues that came up from this research. I am glad that a lot of my work has been published in book chapters and journals. I have also presented the findings of this research at various local and international conferences.

In addition, together with a student at St Paul's and with the financial support from Ecumenical HIV and AIDAs Initiative for Africa (EHAIA), we initiated a course on Gender, Sexuality, Theology and HIV and AIDS that has been rolled out to members of the Sudan Council of Churches – targeting men and women church leaders. Recently, I was appointed Director, Centre for Parliamentary Studies and Training (CPST) Kenya where I hope the issues in this book will be brought to the foreground.

I am grateful for the opportunities to have taken the debate on gender, religion and sexuality to a larger audience, both through this book and through face to face interaction during trainings and in academic conferences. To all who read this book, my hope is that personal issues of women will slowly but surely find their rightful place in workplaces.

Prof. Nyokabi Kamau
NAIROBI, FEBRUARY 2013

Acknowledgements

To complete this work I received love and support from very many people, all of whom I am deeply indebted. My most sincere gratitude goes to the Gender Equity in Commonwealth Higher Education (GECHE) project headed by Prof. Louise Morley for funding my doctoral studies which culminated in this book.

Thanks also to Dr Anne Gold, my doctoral supervisor, for being my teacher and my friend; for introducing me to women's studies and for always seeing the person behind the PhD. I have continued to benefit enormously from Anne's invaluable support and encouragement even post-PhD.

I thank the late Prof. Diana Leonard and Dr Marianne Coleman for reading drafts of the PhD work on which this book is based, Prof. Elaine Unterhalter who read the full first draft of the book and gave very useful comments, and Prof. Jane Onsongo, Dr Gichure and Dr Chege Githiora who read drafts of this work and gave invaluable comments. Thanks also to Jeremy Nga'ngá who edited this entire revised edition.

Thanks to Prof. Michael Kelly whom I first met through his inspiring writings on HIV and AIDS in African universities. While he was not officially involved in my doctoral studies, he provided great encouragement, academic advice, and support. Prof. Kelly also kindly agreed to write the foreword to this book.

To Nick Mulhern and Dorothy Garland of the Association of Commonwealth Universities, Masimo, Kuyok Abol, Irene and all my dear friends in London and Nairobi who have supported me throughout this journey, I say a simple thank you. I also say thank you to my very supportive group of women friends, 'Valentines', for their prayers and encouragement.

I thank my parents Mr and Mrs Kamau Njongeri, my siblings, Njoki, Wangui, Wairimu, Muthoni, Mbaire, Waiganjo, Washuka and Wambui, and all my nieces and nephews for their love and prayers. Thanks also go to all my house helps who have always ensured that my home is well managed in my prolonged absences. And thanks to all the women and men who participated in this study.Unfortunately, the need to use pseudonyms to maintain anonymity means I cannot thank them by their names. However, their stories provide the backbone of this work.

Special thanks to my children Mugane and Mumbi, and my husband Mundia, for their unwavering love and support. And to my last daughter Wanjiku, born after the PhD and who has been my great source of inspiration for my work. It is my sincere hope that she grows up in a world where justice and equality are the core norms.

Abbreviations and Acronyms

ACU	-	AIDS Control Unit
ACU	-	Association of Commonwealth Universities
AIDS	-	Acquired Immune Deficiency Syndrome
ART	-	Antiretroviral Therapy
ARVs	-	antiretroviral drug(s)
BERA	-	British Educational Research Association
CHE	-	Commission for Higher Education
FAWE	-	Forum for African Women Educationalists
GECHE	-	Gender Equity in Commonwealth Higher Education
HIV	-	Human Immunodeficiency Virus
ICL	-	I Choose Life
JKUAT	-	Jomo Kenyatta University of Agriculture and Technology
MDGs	-	Millennium Development Goals
NACC	-	National AIDS Control Council
UNAIDS	-	Joint United Nations Programme on HIV and AIDS
UNESCO	-	United Nations Educational Scientific and Cultural Organisation
UNISA	-	University of South Africa
VCT	-	voluntary counselling and testing
WCC	-	World Council of Churches
WMHE	-	Women and Management in Higher Education

Abbreviations and Acronyms

= 1

Background and Setting the Scene

> *Our days begin to end the day we become*
> *silent about things that matter."*
>
> Martin Luther King

Introduction

According to Stephen Lewis, the UN envoy to Africa, the Acquired Immune Deficiency Syndrome (AIDS) is viewed as the 'biggest practical and moral challenge facing the world' (Lewis, 2003). The 3rd and 6th Millennium Development Goals (MDGs) focus on promoting gender equality, women's empowerment, and halting and reversing the spread of HIV and AIDS, malaria and other diseases. The inclusion of HIV and AIDS and gender equality in the MDGs suggests the importance they have been given internationally. Gender equality has been seen to be one of the ways that will help to halt the spread of HIV and AIDS as noted in a speech by Lewis (2003):

> The toll [of AIDS] on women and girls is beyond human imagining; it presents Africa and the world with a practical and moral challenge, which places gender at the centre of the human condition. The practice of ignoring a gender analysis has turned lethal.

Lewis argues that a gender analysis in HIV and AIDS policy and programming should be given priority. However, this has not been put into practice in Kenyan universities as I have investigated in this study and the literature reviewed. In the context of HIV and AIDS, gender analysis is a tool that 'uses sex and gender as a way of conceptualising information' (Commonwealth Secretariat, 2002:12). Through a gender analysis, the nature and social realities, life expectations, and economic circumstances of men and women are clarified. In addition, a gender analysis in the area of HIV and AIDS 'provides a framework for analysing and developing policies, programmes and legislation for conducting research and data analysis' (Commonwealth Secretariat, 2002: 12).

My Interest

My interest in this study was to explore the situation in Kenyan universities where it seemed that AIDS and gender issues, especially as they affect senior women staff, were unrecognised (Garland, 2001). By 'senior' I mean women who held academic positions at lecturer level, or administrators as deputy human resource managers, deputy registrars, librarians and other similar positions that would not fall under the category of support staff.

I wanted to carry out a study that could help reveal senior women's experiences with HIV and AIDS in Kenyan universities. I chose to explore women's experiences in order to show how women are silently carrying an emotional, economic and caring burden, when affected by HIV and AIDS (see Chapters Five and Seven). This study suggests that, although HIV and AIDS are not usually associated with well-educated women in Kenya, they too suffer similar silence and burdens to those in the lower social economic status (see also further in the present chapter).

The use of universities as the sites of my study helps to illustrate that even though, as centres of academic excellence, they are expected to lead in making positive changes, this has not been fully achieved as far as gender equality and issues affecting women are concerned. In this study, by using HIV and AIDS, I show that women's personal experiences affect their public and professional lives.

Throughout this book, I have used the term 'affected' to refer to persons whose close relatives have been infected by HIV, or have suffered from AIDS. Such persons' lives become directly influenced by HIV infection and its emotional, psychological and sociological ramifications (UNAIDS, 2004a). All the women in this study were 'affected' because some of their close relatives and friends had suffered from AIDS, many of whom had died by the time I interviewed them.

The term 'infected' is used to refer to those individuals who have had a blood test yielding an HIV positive result. They are generally referred to as 'HIV positive' (ibid.). There are some people who are both infected and affected. In this study, I only asked women if they were affected. However, some of them may also have been infected, but I did not enquire about it because I thought such a question could silence them in ways that would have made the interviews difficult to progress (see Chapter Eight).

My Objectives

My objectives in carrying out this study were to:

- Provide another example of silences, absences and invisibilities of women's personal and private experiences in the workplace (Kenyan universities), using HIV and AIDS as an example.

- Carry out a study that would look at women and see them in ways that traditional social science research does not. To provide a forum where university women's experiences with HIV and AIDS (a condition not usually associated with them), could be listened to and heard.

- Carry out a study that would help me to develop a language and set of theories to work with, which can help to describe women's experiences and reality of their lives.

- Provide a framework through which the management of Kenyan universities could begin to see the need to put in place systems that embrace individuals as whole human beings, where workplace caters for both their private and personal lives.

- Make use of the interviews as a tool for the women to be reflexive* about the factors that may hinder their career progression. This reflexivity, I hoped, would help them to want to 'make a difference' if they were in position to do so.

- Look at whether the AIDS policies and responses in two Kenyan universities had acknowledged that men and women would require different policy responses given the existing gender roles and responsibilities in Kenya.

An Overview of Chapter One

In the following section of this first chapter, I have provided the global and Kenyan statistics on AIDS. I have then provided the global background to draw a picture of the extent to which AIDS has been experienced in the wider context before showing its impact in Kenyan universities. I was not able to get any statistics from the universities on the impact on staff because it was not available at the time. I therefore provide a brief discussion regarding the silence that surrounds HIV and AIDS and its impact on senior staff in the context of African and Kenyan universities. This is followed by a summary of my personal experiences as someone affected by HIV and AIDS. I explain how these experiences have informed my research question. Use of my experiences as part of this study (reflexivity) was informed by a feminist theoretical perspective, which I discuss in Chapter Five. From this background, I state the main research question and the sub-questions. I end the chapter with an overview of the entire thesis.

---

* To be reflexive is where the researcher makes themselves a visible part of the research process. Reflexivity requires that the researcher starts with an awareness their values and how they relate to those being researched.

HIV and AIDS in the Global and Kenyan Context

The United Nation AIDS programme releases annual updates on HIV and AIDS. The 2011 AIDS update shows that by the end of 2010, the total number of people living with HIV globally stood at 34 million. Of these, 50% (about 17 million) were women, with a higher proportion in sub-Saharan Africa (59% of all people living with HIV) (UNAIDS, 2011: 6). An estimated number of 2.5 million children under 15 years of age were living with HIV in 2009 (UNAIDS, 2010a: 23). In the year 2010 alone, there were a total of 2.7 million new infections (UNAIDS, 2011: 7). Despite improved access to antiretroviral treatment and care in many regions of the world, AIDS still claimed 1.8 million lives in 2010 (UNAIDS, 2011: 11). By that time, sub-Saharan Africa remained the most affected by this pandemic as it was home to 22.9 million people living with HIV, which was almost three million less than in 2005 (UNAIDS, 2011).

In Kenya, HIV prevalence stood at 6.2 per cent in 2011 (NACC and NASCOP, 2012: 6). There were about 1.6 million infected adults, 0.95 million of them women aged 15-49 years. It is estimated that in Kenya, in the year 2009, about 49,000 adults and children died from AIDS complications (NACC and NASCOP, 2012), a sharp drop from the figures recorded in the years 2002–2004, when an estimated 130,000 people died each year. New infections had also dropped to around 91,000 in 2011 and the number is expected to decline to about 82,000 in 2013 (NACC and NASCOP, 2012). The majority of these new infections are said to occur among the youth, especially young women aged 15-24 years and young men under the age of 30 years. Nevertheless, the AIDS pandemic threatens to reverse the developmental gains that Kenya has made since independence in 1963 (Nyutho et al. 2005).

AIDS pandemic is not just about the sheer numbers of infected and affected individuals. Rather, it is about lost lives, shattered communities and spiralling developmental crises. Perhaps for this reason, the UNAIDS Executive Director, Peter Piot, acknowledges that this "epidemic will defeat us unless there is an exceptional response from world leaders and publics" (Piot, 2005).

However, this global acknowledgement about the magnitude of HIV and AIDS as a major problem has not been without its contradictions. Parker and Aggleton (2003), for example, argue that although for over two decades countries all over the world have struggled to respond to this epidemic, "issues of stigma, discrimination and denial appear to have been poorly understood and often marginalised within national and international programmes and responses" (p.13). They associate this persistent contradiction to lack of a conceptual and theoretical framework through which people can understand HIV and AIDS-related stigma and its effects. The findings of this study help to make known issues of stigma and discrimination as they affect women in two universities in Kenya. The terms silence, stigma, shame, and denial are commonly used in AIDS discourse and I use them repeatedly in this book. In Chapter Nine, they are discussed in greater detail.

Universities in Sub-Saharan Africa and the AIDS Challenge

The contradiction mentioned in Parker and Aggleton (2003) above on the global scene seems to echo the context of African universities as well. Although the universities have conducted research and acted as advisers to their governments and non-governmental organisations (NGOs), they have continued to act as though the pandemic does not exist in their midst. My readings (e.g., ACU and DFID, 2001; CHE and UNESCO, 2004; Kelly, 2003b; Nyutho et al., 2005; Owino, 2004) and the findings of this study, show that attitudes of denial and AIDS-related stigma continue to plague many African universities (see Chapters Eight and Nine).

Prior to 1999, only a few African universities had shown any worthwhile response to HIV and AIDS (Kelly, 2001). In 1999, the Association of Commonwealth Universities became involved in providing leadership in this area of HIV and AIDS. In 2000, the Association for the Development of Education in Africa (ADEA) working group of the World Bank commissioned case studies of seven African universities to establish the impact of the pandemic on these universities and the responses that each of them had adopted. These universities included Nairobi and Jomo Kenyatta University of Agriculture and Technology (JKUAT) in Kenya, and the Universities of Zambia, Botswana, Namibia, Ghana and Western Cape (in South Africa). All these studies showed that HIV and AIDS were still surrounded by silence and stigma (Anafri, 2000; Chilisa et al., 2001; Kelly, 2001; Magambo, 2000; Nzioka, 2000). The findings of my study suggest that silence and stigma contribute to the inaction about the effects of HIV and AIDS to senior women staff in the two universities, as I show in the data chapters (Seven to Nine).

None of the studies mentioned above point out the need to have responses in place towards staff needs or even a need for being gender sensitive. This was despite the fact that it has become apparent that HIV and AIDS worsens the already existing gender inequalities in all development sectors (Commonwealth Secretariat, 2002). It is notable that in order for African universities to deal with this pandemic, they need to become more open about its impact, and to discourage the secrecy and shame that enshrouds the disease (Francis and Francis, 2006; Kelly, 2001, 2003b). In addition, it has been suggested that Sub-Saharan African universities need to recognise the gender implications of HIV and AIDS not only among the student community, but also among senior staff (Garland 2001). Universities have serious gender inequalities at senior levels as shown by several studies (Kanake, 1995; Lund, 1998; Morley et al., 2005; Onsongo 2000; Singh, 2003; Teferra and Altbach, 2004), and as I discussed in Chapter Six. The non-recognition of the association between gender issues and HIV and AIDS prompted my interest in this study.

HIV and AIDS in Kenyan Universities

Kenyan universities have been affected by the AIDS epidemic. As far back as year 2000, some universities like the University of Nairobi were recording an average of two deaths per week, none of which were publicly associated with AIDS (Nzioka, 2000). As citadels of knowledge and excellence, universities are expected to depict best practices in all their undertakings and are often looked upon as models and pacesetters for the rest of society (Bahemuka and Van der Vynckt, 2001; Morley, 2003a). Unfortunately, this has not been the case as regards HIV and AIDS (Nyutho et al., 2005). Literature available on the disease in Kenyan universities indicates that little information has been documented on the prevalence and impact of the pandemic among university staff (Magambo, 2000; Nyutho et al., 2005; Nzioka, 2000; Owino, 2004). The few reported activities on HIV/AIDS mitigation are mainly concentrated on the student community.

Since the year 2000, the Kenya National AIDS Control Council (NACC) and the AIDS Control Unit (ACU) of the Commission for Higher Education (CHE), have been instrumental in setting up AIDS Control Units (ACUs) in all universities in Kenya. Nyutho, who was involved in creating the ACU curriculum, observes: "Today, the curriculum is gathering dust in a lot of government ministries, including universities, for no apparent reason" (Nyutho et al., 2005: 12).

Even with the setting up of ACUs in Kenyan universities, no study had looked at how senior women were coping with the challenges brought about by HIV and AIDS. I understand that my study is the first one to use women's experiences with this pandemic to provide an example about women's lives and how they remain unrecognised in the workplace. In this study, I have used the experiences of senior women staff in two Kenyan universities, aware of the criticisms that such method may receive in terms of inappropriate data (Clandinin and Connelly, 1998). However, as Clandinin and Connelly (1998) argue, social science is concerned with humans, their relations with themselves and their environments. Social science is therefore founded on the study of experience. Clandinin and Connelly (1998) also point out that in the study of experience it is the researcher who defines the starting and stopping points. The researcher has therefore to be reflexive throughout the study so as not to lose track from huge volumes of data (I discuss reflexivity in Chapter Three). My own experiences guided me on the starting and end points during the conversations with the participants.

In the following sections, I provide a brief discussion on the use of autobiographies and personal experiences in a research. I also explain the reasons I decided to include my own experiences in this thesis.

The Autobiography of the Research Question

The use of researchers' own experiences to locate how a research question or interest in a certain topic is developed is a common feature amongst feminist researchers (Blackmore, 1999; Burke, 2002; Lewis, 1993; Merrill, 1999; Ribbens, 1998; Skeggs, 1994). However, the use of one's experiences as a basis for asking certain research questions but not others is not without problems. There are, indeed, some feminist researchers (e.g., Kelly et al, 1994) who have argued that a researcher need not have experienced something in order to study it.

Research methodologists like Cosslett et al. (2000) have wondered as to what exact extent we can rely on our memories of our own experiences, since memories are subjective and selective. Some of the questions which I ask myself include: How can I justify what can be remembered and why? Are our memories an accurate representation of what actually happens? Certainly, there is the question of what we choose to disclose and feel safe to talk about and what we leave out, and therefore whether dependence on memory is a valid way of generating knowledge.

Although I do not have straight answers to these questions, experiences from other feminist researchers has given me some degree of confidence to work with women's experiences and my own as a valid way of generating knowledge (e.g., Ciambrone, 2003; Du Bois, 1983; Morley, 1999; Onsongo, 2005).

Having considered the above questions, I find it necessary to note the dilemma of sharing my experiences since this involves talking about other people in my life. I am writing about my experiences as someone affected by HIV and AIDS, which naturally means referring to the HIV status of others. The questions I need to address regarding these dilemmas include the following: "What right do I have to publicly write about the lives of others? Is it ethical for me to write about other people without their permission on an issue surrounded by a lot of stigma? " Birch and Miller (2000) observe that some of the ethical dilemmas of doing qualitative research include some tensions, which are not always addressed in formal ethical guidelines. Campbell (2003: 110), for example, documents the case of a woman who declared publicly that she was HIV-positive in a South African township, where the stigmatisation and denial led to her being stoned to death. Similarly, in a small town in Kenya, in April 2006, an HIV positive orphan was hacked to death by his uncle because he could not live with the shame (Ndirangu, 2006).

My view is that it is only in the sharing of people's lived experiences that the private challenges especially those that face women can find space in public policy. Therefore, I made the decision to use experiences (mine and women participants' as valid data in my research).

In the present study, I have argued that in order for Kenyan universities' responses to HIV and AIDS to include women's experiences, it is necessary that these experiences are made public. Moreover, it would be more unethical not to state the personal experiences that elicited my interests in this study (Skeggs, 1995). For ethical reasons, I use the general term of 'relatives' rather than being specific about the people whose lives I write about. Given that I have lost several of my relatives, both close and distant, without any public knowledge of what killed them, it would thus be difficult for those reading my work to associate the information with any one of them in particular.

In addition, the feminist nature of this study provides me with the space to write about sensitive matters. Other feminist researchers (e.g., Chapman, 2003; Doucet and Mauthner, 2002; Mauthner, 1998, 2000; Parr, 1998; Ribbens, 1998; Steedman, 1986) have included their own experiences, which touch on other people's lives and have justified their use as necessary for doing feminist research. Moreover, as the literature and the findings of this study suggest, talking and creating a tolerant and supportive attitude to those affected and infected by HIV and AIDS can help in reducing the challenges of stigma and denial associated with the epidemic (Gichure, 2006).

How my Personal Experiences Informed the Research Question

AIDS creates unique challenges to individuals, communities and whole nations (Barnett and Whiteside, 2002). Through my personal involvement of caring for people I loved, witnessing them die, and seeing my female relatives suffer as they looked after their dying children and husbands, I realised that AIDS was neither just a medical problem nor only for immoral people, as I had believed before I became affected.

In one case where a male relative was sick in the final stages of AIDS, I witnessed the pain his wife went through while caring for him after he suffered a stroke. Despite being sick herself, and having lost two of her children to AIDS, this woman provided 24 hours of care to her husband; he was bedridden, having been discharged from hospital. The only help she received was from her female relatives who could spare some time. I recall one time when another of my infected relatives was admitted for about three months in a public hospital and family members (mainly women) had to go there in turns to help with cleaning him, washing his clothes and feeding him. These experiences made me see that AIDS is indeed a pandemic that has a unique impact on women.

In the university where I worked, there was no talk about HIV and AIDS, at least not amongst staff. Many people behaved as though the problem did not exist at all. There were whispers going around that so and so was unwell, or that people from other universities were dying. The causes of these deaths were, however, not linked to AIDS directly, a point noted in literature on AIDS in Africa (Chilisa et al., 2001; Esu-Williams, 1995; Kelly, 2003a, 2003b; Magambo, 2000; Nzioka, 2000). Indeed, I did not discuss my pain and sorrow with colleagues apart from my head of department who would kindly allow me to rush to hospital whenever the need arose. Given that I had these experiences while working in the university, my work and career development were affected. This was because I spent a lot of time either providing care or comforting those affected. In some cases I helped with fundraising, arranging and attending funerals, among other chores.

Why I Focused on Senior Kenyan University Women

The thought that I may have been the only one in the university suffering silently changed in the year 2002. In that year, I was involved in the process of planning and facilitating a regional workshop on women and management in higher education in Nairobi. The workshop was attended by a group of 25 senior women academics and administrators from 16 universities in the Eastern African region.

While facilitating one of the sessions in the workshop, I talked about my experiences on how HIV and AIDS had affected me. I noted how I spent a lot of my time providing care and support for relatives who were infected or affected. I talked about the impact this had had on my private life and career. I also narrated how trying to maintain a balance between my private life and my career had become a big challenge on my time, financially and emotionally. It emerged that many of the women present had similar experiences. It was clear from the number of women who 'whispered' to me after the session that they had found no space before to talk about such personal issues. This was an indication of what M. J. Kelly (2003b) calls the 'loud silence' surrounding the HIV and AIDS pandemic, especially for women who already are both a silent as well as silenced group. The feminist theorising of the concept of silence is discussed in Chapter Five and the theme comes through in the entire study.

After the above-mentioned workshop, I began to think about this group of women working in universities and how they (like me) were going through experiences that were not only a challenge to their private lives, but also to their careers. I felt that there was a need for intervention especially with regard to senior staff. On silence in universities, Kelly (2003b) notes that, "In their naive belief that they are responding effectively to the epidemic, many institutions have regarded HIV and AIDS as essentially a health problem and a student problem" (p. 2).

I was concerned by the realisation that the social impact of this epidemic on senior staff was not visible in the university community. A similar concern has been echoed in the context of South African universities (Phaswana-Mafuya and Peltzer, 2006).

At the time of conducting the research (2005), I was not aware of any AIDS prevention, care, treatment or support programmes that were specifically targeting staff members. Of particular concern for me was the role played by women in providing care for family members. In many countries that have been ravaged by HIV and AIDS, those of 'high social status' look at the pandemic as a problem for 'others' as noted by Baylies and Bujra in Zambia and Tanzania, (2000), Campbell in South Africa (2003), Kaleeba and Ray in Uganda (1997), and Ochola-Ayayo in Kenya (1997). Writing on the AIDS and economic crisis in the Democratic Republic of Congo (DRC), Schoepf (1997) notes that the tendency of associating

AIDS with prostitution, and low class and morally loose women has hindered prevention amongst the educated women. Indeed, in my five years as a university lecturer then, I did not come across about any initiative that was concerned with experiences of the learned or well-off people in society. Nevertheless, many women have to deal with daily challenges related to the pandemic. Morley (2003b), for example, notes that gender, higher education and HIV and AIDS have not been integrated, leading to a silence in terms of policy, literature and research studies. Like Morley I too saw that there was a need for research integrating these three areas.

I began to reflect on how it would be useful to carry out a study that could investigate whether other universities (not just the one where I worked) had done anything that had taken into consideration the multiple roles that female employees play in the era of AIDS. Even though they are full-time employees, women have other demands. These include looking after the sick at home, coping with HIV and AIDS in their own personal lives, holding a family together and being there to counsel and support bereaved or affected family members (see Chapter Seven).

My study in this book focuses on a group of women who would be considered to be of a higher social economic status. I framed the study within a feminist perspective, which I discuss in Chapter Five. I chose to work with this group of women aware of the argument by hooks (2000) that feminism in the United States did not emerge from the women who were most victimised by sexist oppression, women who had continued to be the silent majority. hook's (2000) concern is that much of the American feminism has tended to focus on the plight of a select group of women, the middle and upper class "housewives, bored with leisure, with the home, with children, with buying products, who wanted more out of life" (p. 1). Hence, when I argue about the challenges facing a group of women who would be considered as better-off (economically and socially) and also highly educated, compared to the majority of Kenyan women who live on less than a dollar a day, I risk being viewed as ignoring the hard realities facing the poor Kenyan women.

However, this study does not claim to be representing the plight of all women in Kenya. This is the reason I have stated that my focus is on a particular group of women who are not viewed as being as much affected by the HIV and AIDS pandemic as the majority poor and uneducated women (Lipinge et al., 2004; Marcus, 1993; VSO, 2003). AIDS has presented some unique challenges different from those hooks (2000) and the feminist movement had to deal with several years ago. Some of these challenges of silence, denial and stigma have been found to continue fuelling the epidemic (see Chapter Nine).

Research Questions

Having reviewed literature on gender, HIV and AIDS and higher education, and from the pilot study, attending conferences on the impact of HIV and AIDS on Kenyan universities (see Chapter Four) and from my own experiences (as I have noted above in the present chapter), I came up with the main research question of this study: Are senior women's experiences with HIV and AIDS taken account of in the ways two Kenyan universities have responded to the pandemic both in policy and programming? Experiences are used in this thesis to refer to the lived responsibilities and challenges that senior university women have to deal with when affected by HIV and AIDS.

In an earlier section in this chapter I have explained why I chose to focus on senior university women. In Chapter Three, I provide a detailed account of the research design, explaining the rationale used in selecting the two universities and the actual research participants that were included in the study.

In order to understand women's experiences within the university structures, it was important to establish their status within the university management. I needed to find out the causes of the silence and invisibilities of university women's voices in the AIDS discourse and workplace policies and practices. The literature reviewed and the findings of this study have shown that AIDS-related silence and stigma in the universities may contribute to lack of policies and responses that take women's experiences into consideration. Therefore, to address all the issues in my research problem I came up with the following questions:

- How are senior women in Weruini and Holy Ghost Universities affected by HIV and AIDS?

- How have the two universities responded to the impact of HIV and AIDS on their senior women staff?

- How does sexuality-related stigma contribute to the inaction and silence about HIV and AIDS amongst university staff (especially among senior women?)

- What suggestions do the women have for improving practices in their universities to make them more accommodating to women's experiences?

An Overview of the Book

This book contains my doctoral research on the experiences of Kenyan women regarding HIV and AIDS that I submitted to the University of London (UK). One of my UK-based examiners advised me to set aside a chapter providing some historical and social-political background of the women that this study targeted for the sake of readers outside Kenya. It was for this reason that Chapter Two was introduced.

A feminist perspective is used throughout the book to study the experiences of women concerned with HIV and AIDS. In Chapter Five, I explain my understanding of feminist perspectives and other concepts that run through the entire data analysis chapters

(Six to Ten). A separate literature review chapter is not included, but literature is used to explain and describe the data throughout the thesis.

My methodology is discussed in two chapters. Chapter Three describes the design that was followed, while Chapter Four specifically focuses on the ethical challenges I faced when carrying out a study that I considered sensitive. While searching for readings on sensitive topics, I was struck by the scarce literature on this area, especially in Kenya. It was for this reason that I set aside an entire chapter for this important issue in my study. I have also noted the scarcity of feminist literature from Kenya, especially one that links women with HIV and AIDS. Consequently, this study draws much on feminist literature from the West. However, Chapter Two draws heavily on writings from Kenya, while the data chapters use both Western and African literature. One of the contributions made by this study is indeed the addition of the voices of Kenyan university women in the AIDS debate, thus intersecting gender, higher education, and HIV and AIDS. What follows is a synopsis of each of the Ten Chapters.

Chapter One outlines the basic contexts to this study and raises some of the issues that I have grappled with. It provides an overview of the global problem of HIV and AIDS. This is followed by some statistics of AIDS, globally and in Kenya. A brief discussion concerning silence about HIV and AIDS and its effect on senior staff in African and Kenyan universities is presented. The chapter then briefly explores the use of experiences and memory in research. The use of my experiences as the researcher is also discussed. This is followed by a summary of the main research question and the sub-questions that I have sought to answer in this study.

Chapter Two explores the social-economic and political context in which Kenyan women find themselves operating. This background focuses on issues that affect women in order to provide a picture of the roles and expectations that Kenyan society has put on women. This is done while focusing on gender relations during colonial rule and the changes that have taken place in Kenya since independence. The aim of this chapter is to provide readers, who are not familiar with Kenya, with an image of the issues affecting women. In order to understand women's experiences with HIV and AIDS, which provide the main data of this study, I summarise the issues that seem pertinent to the women participants. These include: male domination, marriage and family, gender and HIV and AIDS, religion and conflict between the modern/Christian/ Western values and the African traditional values.

Chapter Three explores the methodological processes, theories and practices that I followed in my study. Throughout that chapter, I try to be clear about how my location as a feminist academic affected by HIV and AIDS informs my methodological choices and decisions. The chapter also discusses the approaches and methods used in the study, which include the following: case study approach; sample selection and sample size; snowball sampling technique; use of in-depth conversational interviews; focused interviews; the tape recording of interviews; field notes; Weruini policy; issues of validity and reliability; and, data analysis.

During my research on what I consider to be a sensitive topic, I faced many ethical challenges. **Chapter Four** begins by discussing my understanding of ethics and gives an explanation as to why my study qualified to be termed sensitive. A discussion and explanation of the ethical dilemmas I faced during various stages and aspects of my data collection, analysis and dissemination follow. The chapter contains a discussion of the ethical issues that were pertinent in a study of this nature; that is, a woman researching senior men and women on a subject hardly discussed in their circles. The discussion contained in Chapter Four can help and encourage researchers doing a similar type of research.

In **Chapter Five**, the feminist perspective that has guided the study is explained. In this chapter, I provide a brief explanation of why I term my study feminist, although the term raises some controversies amongst some African scholars. Using a feminist perspective, I discuss the themes and concepts, which emerged from both my literature and the interviews. My questions and reading of the data were guided by these concepts. The structure of the thesis follows these themes. They include patriarchy, discourse, 'personal as political', and care.

In **Chapter Six**, I begin to make the voices of the women in my study heard – highlighting the issues that they noted as affecting their status in their universities. I use data from the conversational interviews with the women and figures of the seven senior-most positions in the two universities studied to show the gender disparities in the two universities. The chapter suggests that the gross under-representation of women in senior positions is caused by the failure to recognise the need for adequate policies and practices to protect women's rights. This ensures that women are disadvantaged more than men when faced with challenges like those presented by the AIDS pandemic.

In **Chapter Seven**, data from interviews with women is used to highlight the 'personal as political', while showing the need to consider the personal challenges within university AIDS discourses. The university women's personal experiences with HIV and AIDS (for example pain, anger, guilt, shame, and financial and care responsibilities) are discussed. Means of support and how university women cope with professional and personal demands are also discussed. This chapter looks at ways in which women's experiences can be used as a starting point for including gender in AIDS policies and practices at the workplace.

Chapter Eight discusses the impact of HIV and AIDS on the two universities under study as seen by both the management and the women. It also looks at the responses that the two universities have made in relation to HIV and AIDS. The interviews with both men and women reveal that the two universities were more concerned about the welfare of students, but not staff, especially regarding HIV and AIDS initiatives. I discuss this lack of concern while looking at its implications for women. The chapter also presents a brief analysis of the AIDS policy of one of the universities studied.

Based on the interviews with both men and women in this study, it became apparent that lack of an open discourse on sexuality was contributing to the stigma and silence about HIV and AIDS. In Chapter Nine, I summarise the underlying explanations about silence, stigma, shame and sexuality in the Kenyan context. Using data from interviews, the chapter looks at ways in which the shame associated with sexuality contributes to women's silence and insufficient presence in the AIDS discourse. Some modern cultural and religious beliefs that make AIDS (a disease viewed to be mainly sexually transmitted) shameful especially to women are explored. The persistent silence around AIDS that was apparent in the two universities and how that silence affects the policies and practices that the universities adopt, are also discussed.

Finally, **Chapter Ten** provides a summary of the main findings of this study. In this chapter I also reflect on the limitations of the present study, make suggestions for good practice, point out the contributions this study has made, suggesting areas for further research and an epilogue.

= 2 ========================

The Situation of Women in Kenya: Framing the Context

Introduction

Experiences of senior university women, which form the backbone of this study, need to be understood within the women's wider social, economic and political context. Individual women's experiences are intertwined with their social-cultural and political environment. I focus this chapter on issues that affect women, in order to illustrate the roles and expectations that Kenyan society places on women. Such a background helps to clarify Kenyan women's experiences, which were the focus of this study. Patriarchy, which is deeply entrenched in the Kenyan society, helps to sustain male dominance (Chapter Five has more on patriarchy).

I begin the chapter by providing some brief geographical, historical and political background of Kenya. I then trace the changes that have taken place in Kenya, from the pre-colonial and pre-Christianity period to the current period, and the changing roles of women over time. I explore how these roles dis-empower women. This is followed by a discussion on the situation of Kenyan women, especially with reference to the challenges presented by HIV and AIDS. I move on to examine how the institutions of marriage and religion, which are founded on a patriarchal tradition, contribute to women's powerlessness and silence, especially under the current HIV/AIDS regime.

A Brief Geographical and Historical Background on Kenya

Kenya is in East Africa, lying astride the Equator and bordering the Indian Ocean on the east, between Somalia and Tanzania, Lake Victoria on the southwest, Uganda on the west, South Sudan on the northwest, and Ethiopia on the north. Nairobi is Kenya's capital and the largest city in the country.

As at 2010 census, Kenya's population is estimated at 43,013,341. Of these 99% per cent are people of African origin, divided into about 42 ethnic groups of which the Bantu (Kikuyu, Luyhia, Kamba, and Gusii) and the Luo and Kalenjin speaking Nilotics are the dominant communities. The official language in the country is English, while Kiswahili is the national language (Columbia University Press, 2000). The British colonised Kenya for over 60 years and she was granted her independence on 12 December, 1963. In 1964, the country became a Republic, with Jomo Kenyatta as its first President.

Kenyan Women in the Pre-colonial and Colonial Period

In order to understand the position of Kenyan women in the modern political and economic dispensation, it is necessary to make clear the structures under which they operated before the colonial period and during the colonial era. House-Midamba (1990) argues that the status of Kenyan women deteriorated during the colonial rule. She notes that this deterioration was particularly noticeable because, in the pre-colonial era, "although women were to some extent subordinate to men under the African customary law, in many respects the roles of men and women were complementary in nature" (House-Midamba, 1990: 23).

The pre-colonial Kenyan communities practised subsistence agriculture and some forms of trade, especially in the case of the coastal communities. Production was mainly meant to meet basic needs of food as opposed to profit. Division of labour was mainly based on gender roles (Kenyatta, 1938; Odinga, 1967). While there was division of labour based on gender, studies have shown that in many African communities, women performed between 70 and 80 per cent of the total workload available (House-Midamba, 1990). In addition, there existed gender disparities with regard to access and control of land (House-Midamba, 1990). Land and domestic animals were the main sources of wealth in many communities, while women's access to land was mainly through their husbands or sons (Elkins, 2005). Once married, women were allocated land where they could grow crops for family subsistence. Men had supervisory roles over land since there was no individual ownership as land belonged to the tribe (Elkins, 2005; House-Midamba, 1990). Although women did not 'own' land, they had land user rights and they also played important roles as midwives, and elders of extended families and kinship networks (this was especially for older women). Some were chiefs while others performed ritual duties and were placed in charge of ancestral shrines (House-Midamba, 1990). Women also owned property in the form of livestock such as cattle, goats, chickens and sheep (ibid).

Even though Kenyan women had certain powers in the pre-colonial times, the Kenyan traditional culture was predominantly patrilineal and patriarchal. In this environment, men were the predominant force (Odinga, 1967). When the colonialists took over control of the country, they also emphasised male dominance by transferring men's supervisory rights over land to individual legal ownership (Elkins, 2005). As a result of this individual land ownership, women could be denied access to land, something that was new and foreign (Lovett, 1989). This situation exerted a negative impact on the status of women in property ownership.

While Kenyan women had been denied land ownership and were subjected to the control of men in the traditional society, their conditions were made even worse by the coming of the colonialists. According to Onsongo (2005), colonial laws disrupted and displaced women's gender roles. This was done through the introduction of cash crops, formal education and the monetary economy. The female farming systems already in place were not encouraged by the colonial system. While some men secured employment either in large cash crop farms or as clerks in government offices, many women remained in rural areas producing subsistence food (Onsongo, 2005).

Formal education also became mostly available to men; this meant that the majority of women remained illiterate, and, therefore, could not participate in modern economic transactions (Odinga, 1967). Women's work became classified as non-work since it did not fit into the economic criteria of the colonial system (Onsongo, 2005). This undervaluing of women's work has persisted to present times, creating challenges for women who have to perform duties that continue to be seen as non-work. With HIV and AIDS, the challenges are more serious because it is women who mainly expected to care for the infected, an issue I explore further in Chapter Seven.

Moreover, due to migrant labour that led to many men moving to urban areas, rural families became increasingly female-headed, which forced many women into serious poverty levels hitherto not experienced (House-Midamba, 1990). House-Midamba (ibid) has also documented that colonial state policies limited and controlled women's ability to migrate and work in the urban areas. Female migration from rural to urban areas was a subject of controversy during the colonial times and indeed up to this date. Obbo (1980) notes that women who migrated to urban areas alone were always viewed as problematic by both urban authorities and migrant men; it was seen as a cause of marital instability and a disruption of traditional values (Obbo, 1980).

In the early stages of colonial rule, the government worked to restrict the movement of women, especially unmarried ones. The aim was to keep them in the villages so that men could be encouraged to return home, thereby ensuring a regular supply of labour. This new division of labour seems to have created male breadwinners with women dependent on them, a situation that created a sense of powerlessness amongst women. Such a situation has continued to affect their participation in public decision-making to this day (Onsongo, 2005).

The colonialists also introduced Christianity and formal education, both of which had different impact on men and women. Both (especially girl's education) were originally viewed with suspicion by many of the tribal elders. These elders felt that the presence of colonial officers and missionaries "interrupted a sheltered, isolated, and idyllic life in the villages" (Kanogo, 2005: 6). The movement of girls from villages to the mission schools was initially seen as a way of 'spoiling' the good village girls. There was fear that the daughters of such women would no longer make good wives and mothers. The concern was that education would turn girls into prostitutes. Even with this suspicion, the missionaries managed to have some girls join the mission schools, many of which were located away from the villages. These girls would be boarders; hence, they would spend three months away from their villages, something that had not happened before (Kanogo, 2005).

However, the 'freedom' that came along with mission and colonial education had its contradictions, especially for women. The missions' interest was to produce moderately literate girls steeped in Christian ideals and suitable as wives for Christian men (Kanogo, 2005). The syllabus that the girls were offered in the missionary schools was designed to cultivate their domestic skills for their roles as wives and mothers (Kanogo, 2005). While some girls got jobs as nurses and teachers, "Missions hoped that this would be for about two to three years only before marriage. In the missions, as well as in the villages...women were not expected to combine marriage and careers" (Kanogo, 2005: 203).

The above-mentioned attitudes have continued to affect women's careers and, indeed, the very perception and structure of workplaces (Maathai, 2006). As educated Christians, women are still expected to retain their traditional roles of being mothers and submissive wives, while at the same time opening up new normative spaces for themselves (ibid). Unfortunately workplace norms in Kenya do not allow for combining of domestic and public roles, hence creating conflicts for professional women who try to balance the dual careers (Onsongo, 2005). I explore this issue further in Chapter Seven.

Post-colonial Era

The first decade of independence under Jomo Kenyatta was characterised by disputes among ethnic groups, by economic growth and diversification, and by the end of European dominance. After Kenyatta's death in 1978, Kenya experienced a regime which had limited democracy for 24 years (1978-2002) under President Daniel Moi. These years were marked by a struggle for multiparty democracy, which saw the country go through turbulence and ethnic fighting. Women who tried to campaign for their rights during this period, were often harassed and silenced (Oduol and Kabira, 2000). Forced under the constitution to retire, Moi was succeeded by Mwai Kibaki in 2002.

As at December 2011, the Kenyan Parliament had 222 members, 210 of them elected, while 12 are nominated by political parties represented in Parliament. Of this, 22 (10%) are women, eight of whom were directly elected and the rest nominated. Majority of the nominated seats went to women (10 out of 12), mainly as a move by the political parties to meet a legal requirement that a third of their nominees must be women. This is the highest representation of women in Parliament since independence.

Although this is a big improvement from the previous years where between 1963 and 2002 only 52 women had been elected and 33 nominated and the current numbers still lag far below the required critical mass of at least 40 per cent. With such low representation in Parliament, Kenyan women have been excluded from participation in key governance structures and have been deprived of their basic human rights and access to and ownership of strategic resources especially land (Nzomo, 2003a). However, Nzomo (ibid) argues that with democratic transitions and legal reforms that have been evident in Kenya since the 1990s, gradual political changes have taken place. These changes are evident in the rise, though very small, in the number of women in senior political positions (see also Kamau, 2010).

A male dominated political structure, like the one in Kenya, continues to block any agenda that attempts to address issues affecting women (Kamau, 2003). An example is the Women's Equality and Domestic Violence Bills that have been pending in Parliament for many years because the majority of male legislators may not support the enactment of such laws, which can have a negative effect on them (Kamau, 2003; Nzomo, 2003a). It was only in during the Ninth Parliament that the Sexual Offences Act was enacted, which was as a result of serious lobbying by women inside and outside Parliament under the leadership of Hon. Njoki Ndung'u who was a nominated member (see also Kamau, 2010 for more on value added by women in the 9th parliament).

There are many challenges that have continued to face Kenyan women mainly as a result of their unequal status to men, especially in policy-making. In the sections that follow, I look at some of these challenges.

HIV and AIDS and Gender in the Kenyan Context

Some of the factors that lead to women's vulnerability to HIV and AIDS include social, biological, political, economic and psychological issues (Kamau, 2004a; KANCO, 2000). On the social side where the interests of this study lie, this vulnerability seems to be related to what Gupta, et al. (2003) refer to as 'a dominant ideology of femininity' in many societies, especially those most devastated by HIV and AIDS. These societies cast women in a subordinate, dependent and passive position. In this position, Gupta, et al. (2003) note that virginity, chastity, motherhood, moral superiority and obedience are seen to be key virtues of the ideal woman.

In the era of HIV and AIDS, women are viewed either as transmitters of the virus, or just carers for the sick, or bearers of (un) healthy children (Baylies and Bujra 2000; Campbell, 2003; and Gupta et al., 2003). Literature on HIV and AIDS suggests that the "effectiveness of HIV and AIDS programmes and policies is greatly enhanced when gender differences are acknowledged, the gender specific concerns of women and men addressed, and gender inequalities reduced" (Gupta et al., 2003: 5). HIV and AIDS needs to be understood within the context of other social epidemics 'such as poverty, gender inequality, abuse of children, racism, ethnic conflict, war, international injustice, and discrimination on the basis of sexual orientation' (Dube, 2004: 117). Given that HIV and AIDS thrive within other social epidemics, it is the marginalised members of the world who are more vulnerable to infection and who happen to lack quality care. It is worth noting that being marginalised is not always a problem of the poor and ignorant. Even highly educated people get marginalised because of other factors such as gender, which is the focus of this study.

Gender activists and analysts on issues of HIV and AIDS argue that gender inequality is not just a matter of justice and fairness; it can be fatal in the context of HIV and AIDS (Green, 1996; Gupta et al., 2003; Kamau, 2004a; Mbilinyi and Kaihula, 2000; NACC, 2003; Okello, 2003; Travers and Bennet, 1996; Wood, 2002). In this regard, therefore, Kenyan women need to be enabled to complete their education, perform like men, earn good living wages, achieve relatively autonomous and sustainable livelihoods, and be protected against sexual and other forms of abuse and violence. These include wife beating, sexual harassment at work, wife inheritance and rape. Unfortunately, this has not been easy in an environment that is not always supportive of women, and especially where the leadership has not fully embraced gender issues as they relate to problems like HIV and AIDS (Okello, 2003).

One of the leadership tasks that we are yet to live up to in Kenya is forming of partnerships with people living with HIV and AIDS, an issue that was mentioned by one of the women in this study (see Chapter Ten). These would include providing leadership in disclosure of HIV status among the leaders themselves, taking special account of women, and ensuring that HIV and AIDS is rated high on the public agenda (Gichure, 2006), which brings me to the issue of the stigma that has persisted amongst the well-to-do and high profile people in Kenya.

So far, Kenya has not had any high profile personality going public about their HIV status. The de-linking of HIV and AIDS from those viewed by society as 'important' or highly educated, has affected the ways African universities have responded to the effects of the pandemic on their senior staff (Lindow, 2006; Phaswana-Mafuya and Peltzer, 2006). I explore this further in Chapter Eight. For over two decades now, much of the AIDS debate is still surrounded by theories that sexual promiscuity is to blame for the spread of the pandemic, especially in Africa (Hunter, 2003). The earlier beliefs amongst many Kenyans were that tourists and truck drivers brought AIDS from foreign countries. The idea of blaming and pointing fingers when people are faced with such a disease is not unique to Kenya, as noted by O'Sullivan (1996).

The AIDS debate in Kenya has portrayed men as victims of circumstances, while women are portrayed as the creators of those circumstances, either as prostitutes, or as wives who infect their partners and husbands (Ochola-Ayayo, 1997). Equally, there have been several debates over why there are more AIDS cases in Africa than anywhere else in the world (Arnfred, 2004; Barnett and Whiteside, 2002; Hunter, 2003; Sarpong, 2005; Vliet, 1996). Of interest to my study was the fact that a number of these arguments have tended to blame African women (Hunter, 2003). The findings of this study suggest that the linking of AIDS to promiscuity of women seems to cause stigma and silence, especially amongst educated and Christian women who would not want to be associated with such a disease.

Ochola-Ayayo (1997), for example, notes that polygamy has been cited as a cause of promiscuity among women. He argues that young women in polygamous relations would seek sexual satisfaction outside the marriage that their older and weaker husbands could not provide. This model portrays men either as husbands or casual partners who are often innocent victims who get infected by their unfaithful wives or girlfriends. I discuss the discourse of blame in Chapter Nine.

This blaming of women has also been noted by Campbell et al. (2006) in a study in South Africa:

> Many of our informants spoke of the way in which 'the weakness of women' fuelled the epidemic, insisting that it was women rather than men who were responsible for promoting sexual morality (despite much evidence for women's relative lack of power in sexual relationships (Campbell et al., 2006: 134).

On blaming women and materialism, Ochola-Ayayo (1997) argues that women do not remain in any friendship with men without material compensation. He notes that, "in Kenya, few women would pay the expenses of an evening out with a man, no matter how rich they might be" (Ochola-Ayayo, 1997: 114). The respondents in Ocholla-Ayayo's study (ibid) noted that women become unfaithful to their husbands in order to earn additional income and other material benefits. Although men were also cited as being unfaithful, it seemed that if there were no single women and prostitutes willing to have sex with men, the men would not become immoral.

In Kenya, men are presented as though they cannot control their sexual urges, while women are expected to control themselves and to avoid tempting men (Chege, 2004; NACC, 2003; Shisanya, 2002). The sexuality discourse and how it perpetuates silence and stigma, especially among the more educated women, is discussed further in Chapter Nine.

The core problem with many behaviour models that have been used in AIDS prevention campaigns is their irrelevance to women. These models have focused on behaviour change, using the popular 'ABC' slogan (A for abstinence, B for being faithful, and C for condom use). The 'ABC' script fails to address the specific needs of women, as they may not always make free choices about their sexuality. In order for people to be in control of their sexuality, they need to be empowered, and sometimes this empowerment cannot just be achieved at individual level as it involves real political and economic empowerment (Ahlberg, 1991; Campbell,

2003). Empowered people have access to symbolic power, which Campbell (2003) defines as perceived respect and recognition from others. Campbell quotes Paulo Freire as having asserted that the development of critical consciousness would contribute to positive behaviour change among marginalised people. This kind of empowerment seems to be lacking among many Kenyan women and girls (Chege, 2004), an issue I return to in chapters where the findings of this study are presented.

AIDS-related stigma is worsened by the fact that many Kenyan employers have not responded to this pandemic as they should. There has been concern that only a few companies provide medical care, counselling and support systems for employees infected or affected. It has also been noted that discrimination against people with HIV persists in the workplace, where many of those infected are rarely promoted or offered opportunities for further training. The findings of this study also show lack of support in the two universities studied, as discussed in the data chapters.

Religion has played its role in the sex-related stigma and indeed in the silence. In the section that follows, I explore how religion has impacted on people's attitude to sexuality and AIDS.

Religion and AIDS Stigma in Kenya

The majority of Kenyans follow three main religions, but there is no state religion. About 78 per cent of the population are Christians, 10 per cent are Muslim, while the rest follow various traditional religions (Association of Commonwealth Universities, 2006: 219). Christianity has greatly influenced people's belief systems in Kenya and it is seen to have a strong impact on people's attitudes and, to some extent, behaviour (Hoehler-Fatton, 1996; Kuria, 2003;Shisanya, 2002).

Reliance on religion during times of crisis is not unique to Kenya as has been noted elsewhere (Cheemeh et al., 2006; Ciambrone, 2003). Kenyan women have learnt to turn to God because they lack other means through which they can question their oppression (Onsongo, 2005). Some studies have shown that women's reliance on God seems to cut across class and education level (for example Kuria, 2003; Onsongo, 2005 and in this study as discussed in Chapter Seven). In his study, Kuria (2003) interviewed six leading Kenyan women authors with the aim of understanding their perceptions, interpretations and experience of gender issues in Kenya and in Africa in general. One of the women writers, (Pat Ngurukie) argued that women should submit to their husbands and that gender equality is like a myth that cannot be sustained. Ngurukie's views on what a good African woman should be are captured in the following extracts:

> In the African context, and I think it is also biblical, a man is always the head of the family...I have never believed that I could be equal to a man just because of my qualifications. In an ideal biblical setting I think there can be a case for you (referring to the male interviewer) being paid more even if we are doing the same job. Spiritually, it goes back to the Bible... you are supposed to be the head of the family (Kuria, 2003: 153).

On what God expects of a woman even when her husband is unfaithful or even abusive, Ngurukie has noted:

> I know what my God has told me to do: 'Wives submit to your husbands and husbands love your wives'... If a woman truly submits to her husband, it is upon the Lord to make the husband love h e r . If only women would say 'Lord we have seen how we have been oppressed, we have tried to bring to the attention of our men ... and nothing is working, we now wash our hands. We, at least, submit to you, the highest authority. Deal with our men'. ...Prayers would change things. And women, be they Western or African, would no longer need to fight for equality...I would advise any woman who has been thrown out by her husband to take heart and stop being bitter and leave everything to God... just forgive (Kuria, 2003: 164-7).

Although Ngurukie's views do not represent all educated women in Kenya, they do give us a glimpse of the Kenyan Christian view of a woman.

Nevertheless, the influence of Christianity does not mean that Kenyan women simply sit back and wait for God to perform miracles in their lives as many of them have engaged in resisting oppression in different ways (Kuria, 2003; Oduol and Kabira, 2000). In the context of HIV and AIDS, however, even women who had learnt to cope with other 'normal' problems may find it difficult to cope with the challenges that the AIDS pandemic presents. Religion has been a source of consolation for many people, especially for women who often are the care-givers of those infected (Smith and McDonagh, 2003). Nonetheless, this support has not been without its contrasts as AIDS has drawn much of its stigma from the Christian view of sexuality, with women being portrayed as the ones who tempt men (Kamaara, 2005).

The AIDS debate is permeated with the Christian views of morality, blaming AIDS on sin and considering it a punishment and plague from God for those who go against His law, as prophesied in the Old Testament (Khathide, 2003; Mbilinyi and Kaihula, 2000). It can be argued that the same Church, although comforting women, also silences them as those in churches may be afraid to talk about their experiences with the epidemic lest they be branded immoral. This was a central issue in one of the universities in this study as I show in Chapters Eight, Nine and Ten.

One contradiction in Kenya is that, although many people adhere to the Christian faith, they also tend to be influenced by the traditions of their tribes (Kamaara, 2005). Given the blending of different cultures and religions that has taken place in Kenya in the last century, it sometimes becomes difficult to understand which one has more influence on the people's attitudes and behaviour. This contradiction between the traditional cultural and the modern Christian context were found in this study to contribute to silence on issues of sexuality (see Chapter Nine). Closely related to religion is the institution of marriage, which I discuss next.

Marriage and Family in Relation to Women's Careers in Kenya

Literature available from Kenya suggests that marriage is seen as compulsory for men and women (CIA, 2005a; House-Midamba, 1990; Kanogo, 2005; Kiluva-Ndunda, 2001; Kuria, 2003; Stamp, 1986). In traditional Kenyan culture, women were taught that marriage was the highest point in their lives only to be surpassed by motherhood. Women's status tended to be ascribed rather than achieved. Thus, their recognition was viewed in terms of daughters, wives and mothers (Lovett, 1989).

One of the important features carried over from traditional to modern Kenya is the importance of marriage and family. The ideal family is still seen as one with a male breadwinner, and a wife is seen as one whose most important duty is to take care of her husband and children (Kuria, 2003; Maathai, 2006). This is seen as a 'value system' that needs to be adhered to as House-Midamba (1990) observes:

> This value system has placed severe restrictions on women in post-independent Kenya. In many cases, women are unable to reconcile the role of being a wife and mother with the ability to participate as wage earners. Many women still believe that females should remain at home and care for their children (p. 127).

In the modern setting, the image of a good respectable woman is still one who is married and has children. Although an educated and well-off woman may delay marriage (entering into it after her mid 20s), it is still seen as an important achievement regardless of the level of education and the position she holds in society (World Bank, 1989).

Studies about Kenyan women's roles in the family (for example, House-Midamba, 1990; Kiluva-Ndunda, 2001; Obbo, 1980; Onsongo, 2005;Stamp, 1986) have shown that women continue to bear the main responsibility for the welfare of families; they provide the physical labour required for domestic responsibilities. While differences exist in the domestic responsibilities played by women of different social classes, rural/urban, educated and not educated, married/single, Kiluva-Ndunda (2001) argues that even middle class women are the principal persons responsible for domestic work:

> A working wife and mother is also responsible for finding another women whom she employs to assist her with domestic work. This means that if the house help leaves, which is often the case, the woman has to arrange for alternative child care until she finds replacement. Consequently, like most mothers in developing countries, mothers in Kenya face tremendous pressure to balance their careers and the traditional homemaker roles. In most cases, this becomes impossible because of the separation between the home and the workplace (p. 18).

The workplace in Kenya is not organised to take account of the various responsibilities of women as wives, mothers, workers, and as members of the extended families and communities (Kiluva-Ndunda, 2001; Onsongo, 2005). Kenyan employers expect a clear separation between the public and the private spheres. Research about Kenyan women's performance in the workplace has shown that this separation of private and public roles limits women's participation in employment (Khasiani, 2000; Kiluva-Ndunda, 2001; Manya, 2000; Onsongo, 2000, 2005; Stamp, 1986). Women's gender roles as wives and mothers have been used to deny them senior positions in the workplace as it is usually assumed that these roles will interfere with their performance (Kamau, 2002; Kiluva-Ndunda, 2001).

Patrilineal sexual division of labour from the pre-colonial and the pre-capitalist societies have been retained in the workplace. There has also been a combination of distorted views of Victorian and Christian notions about male superiority, which has created an image of Kenyan women that reflects inferiority (Kiluva-Ndunda, 2001; Obbo, 1980; Stamp, 1989). For employed women in Kenya, this is a challenge, as their positions are treated with suspicion (Kiiti, 1993).

While on the one hand, an employed woman's income is seen

as an advantage to both her nuclear and extended families, on the other hand, this independence is also viewed as having a negative effect on her marriage and family stability. This ambivalence creates a sense of guilt for many employed women, as they do not feel that they are doing the right thing to stay on their jobs. Many women struggle to balance all the roles, but without a supporting environment, it is not easy for them. Gender roles and workplace policies that do not take these roles into account emerged as relevant for women's careers in this study. This situation has been worsened by the AIDS epidemic which has brought new demands on employed women, as I discuss in Chapters Six and Seven (Kamau, 2004a, 2004b; Shisanya, 2002).

Summary and Conclusion

The challenges facing Kenyan women that I have raised in this chapter show that deep-rooted patriarchal structures and systems continue to keep Kenyan women in the bottom ranks of society. Patriarchy, which this chapter has shown to be evident in almost all sectors of society, contributes to women's silencing and invisibility, translating into gender-blind policies and programmes especially in the area of HIV and AIDS.

In this chapter I have shown that despite the dominance of patriarchy in almost all institutions, Kenyan women have made some significant strides towards their emancipation, which has largely resulted in the rising number of women in political leadership as shown by an increase, though very small, in the number of women parliamentarians. These efforts by women have, however, been weighed down by the fact that Kenyan society is still at a crossroads between African, Christian and Western cultures. This has resulted in contradictions as pertains to seeking appropriate responses to a national challenge like AIDS. Kenyan men have, for example, been said to be happy to hold on to African, Christian and Western traditions that favour them, leaving women baffled because even workplaces are run within the mixture of all these cultures (Kamaara, 2005; Maathai, 2006).

= 3

Methodology and Research Design

Introduction

The importance of describing the methodology is to make known the mechanism applied in producing knowledge and locating the position of the knower. Methodology is the theory of methods which informs the researcher on a range of issues to adopt in a study (Skeggs, 1997). These issues range from 'who to study, how to study, which institutional practices to adopt, how to write and which knowledge to use' (Skeggs, 1997: 17). Methodology therefore comprises a set of rules that specify how research should be approached (Ramazanoglu and Holland, 2002).

In this chapter, I explore the methodological processes, theories and practices that were followed in the research presented in this book. Throughout the chapter, I make clear how my location as a feminist academic and researcher, affected by HIV and AIDS, informed my methodological choices and decisions. I also explain how my experiences, values and attitudes influenced the methodological choices I made to address the research questions of this study.

Feminist Methodology

Feminist methodology refers to any set of methods that empower research participants. In addition, feminist methodology requires the researcher to think differently about the process of doing research. In Chapter Five I explain how a feminist perspective of doing research provides the framework for this study and indeed informs my methodology.

According to Leonard (2001), feminist research is different from other social science research. This is because feminist research has a participatory role and it challenges the experts while trying to give 'voice' to silenced groups (Leonard, 2001). It also seeks to minimise the hierarchy between the researcher and the researched and to maximise the reciprocity.

Feminist research is especially concerned with ethical issues and it is opposed to treating people as research subjects (Leonard, 2001). Du Bois (1983) notes that feminist methodology gives a researcher the power to name those aspects of women's lives that are not always named in other social science researches. Naming in research is what determines or defines the quality and value of what is named while at the same time denying reality and value to that which is never named, never uttered, that which has no name (Du Bois, 1983). This aspect of naming or not naming some aspects of social life is reflected in the silence around HIV and AIDS, and the invisibility of women's needs in universities.

Du Bois (1983), emphasising this silence, further notes:

> This has been the situation of women in the world. And this silence, this invisibility, has been confirmed and perpetuated by the ways in which social science has looked at and not seen women. But in this silence and invisibility is to be found the reality of women, of our lives, our experience, our vision and potential for new understandings and constructions of our world and ourselves. To address women's lives and experience in their own terms to create a theory grounded in the actual experience and language of women, is the critical agenda of feminist social science and scholarship... as we have all looked through the distorted patriarchal lenses and removing these lenses is no simple task. It is sometimes painful and frightening to see the reality, we have to describe what we see in order to make visible the realities of our experience... (p. 108, original emphasis).

Feminist methodology and approaches help the researcher to begin generating concepts about women's experiences. I derived the words silence and invisibility for the title of my research from Du Bois. I wanted to carry out a study that would look at women and see them in ways that traditional social science research does not. The feminist researcher develops a language and theories to work with, which can help to describe women's experiences and reality of their lives.

Feminist research demands that we generate words and concepts that spring from women's actual experiences. Feminist methodology uses methods, approaches and theories that allow for the understanding of ways in which women's experiences are structured in a male dominated world (Blackmore, 1999; Harding, 1991; Kelly, et al., 1994; Maynard, 1994; Phoenix, 1994; Reinharz, 1992; and Stanley, 1990). Choosing the methodology of a study signifies the researcher's beliefs and boundaries which may be held consciously or unconsciously (Appleby, 1994). My choice of feminist methodology was based on my ontological perspective, which is informed by my initial training as a social worker where I developed a strong belief in people, their emotions, experiences and gender identities.

I choose to use feminist methodology, being well aware of the question that exists among feminist researchers as to whether feminist methodology is a distinct perspective. However, some feminist researchers have identified common epistemological concerns in feminist methodology. These include considering gender reflexively, consciousness raising as central to the research, challenging objectivity, non-exploitation of the research subjects, and empowerment through transformation (Appleby, 1994; Birch and Miller, 2002; Blackmore, 1999; Burgess, 1982; Cook and Fonow, 1990; Doucet and Mauthner, 2002; Harding, 1991; Hollway and Jefferson, 2000; Maynard and Purvis, 1994b; Stanley, 1991).

Harding (1987) argues that feminist research makes use of just about all the methods used in social sciences. However, the way feminists carry out their research is strikingly different from general social science. For example, Harding (1987) notes that a feminist researcher listens differently, being careful to get what the research participants think about their lives, they observe behaviour that may not be seen as significant in traditional social science research and when analysing historical records, they seek examples of newly recognised patterns. It is more the epistemology (because they imply theories of knowledge that are different from the traditional ones), (Harding, 1987; Stanley and Wise, 1990) and methodology, rather than the methods that make feminist research distinct (see also Maynard, 1993; Stanko, 1994). Additionally Ramazanoglu and Holland (2002) note that "feminist methodology is distinctive to the extent that it is shaped by feminist theory, politics and ethics and is grounded in women's experiences" (p. 16).

In addition, Stanko (1994) notes:

> I do not believe that there is a feminist research perspective. I personally rely upon intensive interviews and ethnography as my methodology mainstays. I work from a perspective, which asserts that, women's voices as different as they are from each other converge into some common themes. I call my approach feminist because I believe women's experiences of the world, their knowledge-base and their interpretations are fused within a gendered context. And this context is one of subordination, by and large, to men and to men's needs (p. 96).

Using Stanko's observation, one can assert that it is not just the methods that make feminist research distinct, but the kind of questions asked, how they are asked and the theory guiding each step. All these steps need to take on board feminist ideals that are grounded on women's experiences. Reflexivity is also a key tenet of feminist methodology and I was reflexive as I show below.

Reflexivity

To be reflexive is where the researcher makes themselves a visible part of the research process. Reflexivity requires that the researcher starts with an awareness of their values and how they relate to those being researched. According to Doucet and Mauthner (2002), being reflexive goes:

...beyond the call for the location of the research. It involves transparency and accountability about the theoretical, epistemological and ontological assumptions that influence and inform our knowledge construction (p. 139).

Reflexivity as a methodological strategy is seen as a central tenet in feminist research as argued by several feminists (for example Burke, 2002; Davies, 1993; Hall, 1996; Marshall, 1994; Mason, 2002; Mauthner, 1998, 2000; Morley, 1999; Parr, 1998; Ramazanoglu and Holland, 2002; Stanley and Wise, 1993; and Ulin et al. 2002). It is ethically and politically right for feminists to lead the way in explaining the ways in which research is produced and lived by those producing it (Maynard and Purvis, 1994b). Maynard and Purvis (1994b) further argue that a "focus on autobiographical analysis of what it is like to do research can provide a useful insight into issues often hidden in conventional methodology text books" (p. 1).

In keeping with reflexivity, I have included my own attitudes, values, beliefs and experiences as a university woman, also affected by HIV and AIDS. In feminist research, "the researcher is placed on the same critical plane as the overt subject matter" (Harding, 1987: 9), where it is made explicit how the researcher's experiences have influenced the entire research process. Harding (1987) further observes that, "The researcher appears not as an invisible, anonymous voice of authority, but as a real and historical individual with concrete, specific desires and interests" (p. 9).

I acknowledge that the need to carry out this study has been influenced by my own personal experiences, attitudes, believes and values. As I researched women's experiences with HIV and AIDS, an issue in which I had personal experience, I drew from Shahidian's (2001) experiences when he notes:

I myself, having experienced many aspects of life in exile, did then rely on personal experience as one instrument of my analysis. This background helped me to gain the trust of the interviewees, since informants' awareness of the researcher's close familiarity with the research domain appears to be instrumental in establishing rapport (p. 61).

Reflexivity in feminist research means that the researcher can bring their own values to the research as "it would be impossible not to do so" (Skeggs, 1997: 33). However, one needs to proceed with utmost care and critical attention when trying to produce a valid account.

The conversations I held with many of the women interviewees were made much easier by the common characteristics we shared. These included marital status, age, career experiences, children, extended family obligations, and the fact that we were all affected by HIV and AIDS.

The Case Study Approach

Robson (2002) refers to a case as "the situation, individual, group, or whatever it is that one is interested in' (p.177). In my case, I was interested in an approach that could assist me to describe and explain, for which case studies are best suited (Gillham, 2000a). Gillham (ibid) further argues that a case study can provide a good opportunity for a researcher to understand processes rather than just looking at the end result. A detailed case study helps the researcher to theorise about the wider context (Robson, 2002). The qualitative nature of this study was best suited for a case study approach as it enabled me to describe the experiences of senior university women regarding the AIDS pandemic in detail.

In the broadest application, case studies refer to research that focuses on a single case or single issue, in contrast to studies that seek generalisations through comparative analysis or the compilation of a large number of instances. My choice of the case study approach was based on my belief that research, which intends to illuminate women's experiences, needs to study them in detail, looking carefully at their personal experiences rather than looking for generalisations. Feminist researchers have found that traditional social science may place an emphasis on generalisations, thus obscuring issues and experiences important to particular groups, including women.

The use of case studies is essential in "putting women on the map of social life" (Reinharz, 1992: 164). In deciding to carry out case studies of women within the two selected universities, I believed that women's needs would be defined in their own terms rather than in andocentric and patriarchal terms, as has been the case with much social science research (Reinharz, 1992).

Within the general case study approach, I chose to carry out a set of individual case studies which, as Robson (2002) notes, involve studying a number of individuals with some common features. In order to achieve this objective, I interviewed a total of 20 women in senior academic and administrative positions at two universities, and gathered their experiences about how they were affected by HIV and AIDS. I also sought women's views about how their universities had responded to the epidemic. In addition to the women's stories, I carried out five interviews with senior managers of the two universities under study.

Through the interviews, I was able to establish how the two universities had responded to the AIDS pandemic in terms of their practices, policy and organisational culture. I also used my field notes, observations and AIDS policy of one of the universities (Weruini) as data. I discuss the different methods used in this research later in this chapter.

A Background to University Sector in Kenya

Kenyan universities are divided into two main categories: private and public. In August 2006 (when the shortly after the field work of this research), there were six public universities all of which had been established by an Act of Parliament. The Commission for Higher Education (CHE) regulates both private and public universities. It is a corporate body, which was established by the Universities Act, 1985 Chapter 21 of the Laws of Kenya. CHE has the responsibility for the advancement of university education in Kenya (Owino, 2004). All private universities were established in accordance with the Act, and Legal Notice No. 56, "The Universities Establishment, Standardisation, Accreditation and Supervision Rules".

Besides the public universities, there are also a number of private universities which fall under three categories. The first category includes chartered universities, which are fully accredited by CHE. These were six as at the time of this study. In the second category of private universities are those that operate with Letters of Interim Authority, which allows them to run university programmes, as they await full accreditation from CHE. This category had seven universities at the time of undertaking this research. In the third category are universities that have a Certificate of Registration. There were two universities under this category at the time of research. Appendix Two shows the full list of all the Kenyan universities, their registration status and affiliations as at the time of the study.

Another feature of Kenyan universities is that they fall under either religious or secular categories. The public universities have no religious affiliation, while all except two of the private ones were established by religious bodies, all Christian except one, which has Islamic affiliation. Kenyan universities can, therefore, be said to lie within the public/private/religious category.

I considered this factor in the selection of universities to include in my study where each of these sectors was represented by one university. The two universities selected for this study represented the private/religious and the public categories.

Pilot Study

Before selecting the research participants and commencing fieldwork, I carried out a small pilot study in which I interviewed two men and two women from each of the two universities (Holy Ghost and Weruini). This exercise helped me in two ways: one, checking my research instrument for errors and revising it, and two, paving the way to employ snowball sampling, which I have discussed further below in this chapter.

Selection of Research Participants

Mason (2002) notes that logic is required in qualitative research in the selection of the research participants. This logic should be guided by certain principles and procedures. The first selection I needed to make was the universities to be included in the study. I settled on two out of a total of 19 institutions that had the authority to offer university education in Kenya at the time of study (two universities received Letters of Interim Authority after this study was completed). I chose 'Weruini' for the pseudonym of the public university and 'Holy Ghost' for the private religious university.

The selection of these two universities was based on the fact that they are both large and fairly well established. Holy Ghost, for example, is one of the older and larger religious universities. Besides the fact that nearly all the private universities were affiliated to religious bodies, I sought to know if the responses to HIV and AIDS were different in the two categories. I wanted to see if religion played a role in the attitudes of women and management in Holy Ghost (as I have discussed in a subsequent section). Weruini was selected because it is a well-established public university. In addition, both universities have large numbers of staff, making it possible for me to get an adequate number of women to interview. Some of the newer private universities have small numbers of full-time staff, which could create a problem in getting the right numbers to be interviewed.

For ethical reasons of keeping the cases anonymous, I have changed their names (Wengraf, 2001). I selected only two universities out of the 19 due to the limited resources available to me. The two were not too far from where I live and were also close to each other. Other universities are scattered all over the country, which would have required a lot of resources for travel and accommodation.

The next sampling decision was about the people to be interviewed, including senior women staff and some representatives of management. This was a study about women, although I also interviewed some men managers. Nevertheless, the main participants in my study were women holding senior academic or administrative positions.

I needed to decide on the number of women to interview. An important question one needs to ask about the number of research participants is: "what work do I want my sample to do?" (Mason, 2002: 121). For women participants, I was looking for an adequate number that could help me to gather stories that would illuminate women's experiences. Drawing on the strength of semi-structured, in-depth, and conversational interviews, which I discuss later in this chapter, I carried out a total of 20 interviews; 9 from Holy Ghost and 11 from Weruini. I settled on 20 because of the time and the resources available, and the amount of data that was to be managed from well over 20 hours of conversations. In the following sections, I describe how I arrived at the particular group of 20 women.

Why I focused on Women Only

The focus of my study was to illuminate the silences, absences and invisibilities of women's experiences in universities regarding HIV and AIDS (as I have observed in Chapter One). I thought that listening to women's experiences would help to illuminate much of what had been taken for granted in Kenyan universities' AIDS policies and programming. Indeed, it can be argued that there are times when it is worthwhile to change the story and put women as the centre of analysis (Coleman, 2002; Greed, 1990; Hall, 1996; Stanley and Wise, 1990). It is crucial that women's experiences be brought into the limelight especially in areas where their experiences have not yet been seen as important (Reinharz, 1992). In addition, Reinharz (1992) notes that: "feminist interest in case studies stems from the desire to document aspects of women's lives and achievements for future secondary analysis and the future action on behalf of women" (p. 171).

I also focused on this group of women because, from the literature, there was no evidence of a study that had focused on the experiences of this category of women. I wanted my study to help break the silence that was apparent in the university sector as far as the effects of HIV and AIDS on their senior staff were concerned. The focus, as I have indicated in Chapter One, was on students and support staff who were seen to be more 'at risk' of infection. I could have still focused on men and women, but my intention was to document women's experiences and the same approach I have used can be used to study other groups.

In addition some feminists have noted that women lead lives that have significantly different contours and patterns from those of men (Fogelberg et al., 1999; Humpreys and Gutenby, 1999; Morley, 1999; Probert, 2005; Romanin and Over, 1993). Thus, adapting a feminist methodology can reveal the existence of forms of human relationships, which may not be visible from the position of men (Coleman, 2002; Reinharz, 1992).

By being reflexive (discussed earlier in this chapter) in my methodology, I gave my women participants a chance to experience a sense of 'sameness' with me as the researcher. Burke (2002) observes that this sense of sameness was invaluable in enhancing a relationship of trust with her research participants (see also Kamau, 2001). Nonetheless, it is worth noting that 'sameness' may not always help to generate better data because there can be differences even among people who are socially classified as belonging to the same group (Phoenix, 1994). There were also some differences between my participants and myself that I discuss in Chapter Four.

In addition to women's experiences, I also interviewed four men who represented the management of the two universities. In the next section I discuss how I arrived at the people who participated in this category.

Participants Representing Management

At the time of embarking on data collection, I did not know the number of men or women who would end up in this category of management. I sought to interview people from each of the selected universities who could provide the official position about what the universities were doing regarding HIV and AIDS and I ended up with four men and one woman. The fact that majority of the senior managers were men is an issue I explore further in Chapter Six.

My decision about the number to interview was made during the fieldwork. This was because I was not sure of which people or how many of them would be directly involved in AIDS work before I began the research. There was also the challenge of the availability of senior people to be interviewed. At Holy Ghost, I interviewed two people, one of them the director of the AIDS Control Unit (ACU) who was at the time of the research working alone. He informed me that he was in the process of convening a committee to work with him. The second interviewee at Holy Ghost was a woman who was the deputy human resource manager and her boss (a man) was on leave during the time I carried out my study. I did not manage to interview the Vice Chancellor (VC) of Holy Ghost because he was said to be out of the country during much of my fieldwork period.

In Weruini, I interviewed three people representing management. These included the director of the ACU, the Vice Chancellor, and one professor who was a board member of the ACU. He had special interest in AIDS work and he had been a dean of his faculty. I was unable to reach two Deputy Vice Chancellors (DVCs) in Weruini who I learnt were involved in AIDS work. This was because they were out of the university for much of the time that I carried out the research.

Although I had made some decisions about where to start with the selection of the participants, I maintained an open mind. Robson (2002) notes that in flexible designs, "sampling of who, where, and what does not have to be decided in advance... you need to start somewhere, but the sampling strategy can and should evolve with other aspects of the design" (p. 165). Keeping an open mind was important throughout the selection of my participants as I discuss in the following sections.

Snowball Technique of Selecting Participants

Snowball sampling technique is used when the researcher knows at least one or two participants who fit the characteristics required for the study. Robson (2002) defines the snowball technique as where:

> The researcher identifies one or more individuals from the population of interest. After they have been interviewed, they are used to identify other members of the population, who are themselves used as participants, and so on. Snowball is useful when there is a difficulty in identifying members of the population (p. 265).

The snowball method of identifying research participants can be time consuming and sometimes the contact persons may become unreliable. However, the technique is a good method because it allows one to access participants who may not be easy to identify through 'conventional' methods like letter writing or sending questionnaires' (Standing, 1998).

Due to the sensitive nature of my topic, which is much stigmatised in the places where I was gathering data, and many people fear discrimination especially at the workplace (see Chapter Eight), I settled for the snowballing method to access women participants. An invitation sent through the post, for example, may have been treated with suspicion. People could have thought that the university was involved in the study. In the pilot study, for example, one of the respondents noted that although her university had no explicit policy against hiring HIV-infected persons, there was a mandatory medical examination before one was recruited, and chances were, those infected would not be hired. Thus, an AIDS-related study could still be viewed with some suspicion, hence the use of snowball technique.

During the pilot study, I had a few problems with the snowball technique because the people I originally identified as my contacts turned out to be of no help at all. I had identified one woman and one man to direct me to others affected by HIV and AIDS. I met the woman in a gender conference and we agreed that I would contact her when I was ready to carry out the pilot study. By the time I came back to Kenya, she had been given a senior political position, and had no time to spare for my research. All my efforts to reach her failed. The man did not help either and I discuss this in Chapter Six. Hence, I had to look for other contacts.

Based on these experiences, I decided to work with other contacts and did not rely on the snowball technique as the only method of accessing participants, as I explain later. Experiences of other researchers who have used this technique also helped me to be prepared for changed circumstances (Miller, 1998; Shahidian, 2001). Miller (1998), for example, mentions the problems she encountered from gate keepers who in some cases would influence the kind of responses the interviewees gave. She (ibid) also realised that she was entering a particular network of women. Similarly, Shahidian (2001) notes that use of references to enter into the Iranian exiled community validated his presence and vouched for his trustworthiness. However, there were drawbacks related to him being identified with the political affiliation his references belonged to. In addition, Shahidian explains an incident where one of the reference persons decided to become his spokesman:

> One reference took it upon himself to 'represent' me in the community. He would talk about what he believed I was doing, which did not always represent my intentions ... I noticed that even when I was present, the reference would offer 'clarifications' about my research. Since his comments differed from what I had in mind, I had to redress them. I eventually decided that, valuable though his contacts in the community might be, it was beneficial that I distance myself from him (Shahidian, 2001: 63).

To minimise such situations, I had to work with a group of contact persons from various categories of women. I started off with four women whom I had known before the research (one from Holy Ghost and three from Weruini). Since the decision to interview 20 women had been arrived at before the fieldwork, my intention was to work with the four women to access the rest. My intention was to interview an equal number from both universities, but this became difficult as Holy Ghost turned out to have less number of women senior staff than did Weruini. I also knew only one woman at Holy Ghost, hence, the snowball ended up with five while I managed to approach four directly. Through the initial three women, I was able to access a total of 14 (seven in Weruini and five in Holy Ghost). After interviewing a woman, I would request her to direct me to a colleague in her university. Some directed me while others did not, and that is how I managed to access 14 women participants. In Chapter Four, I provide further discussions of the ethical dilemmas that I had to grapple with in accessing some of these women using the snowball technique.

Because of the challenges I encountered using the snowballing technique, I decided to combine it with approaching potential participants directly as I discuss in the next section. I was also careful that I did not end up with a certain group of women who were friends and therefore with similar characteristics of, for example age, ethnic group, position at university, economic status and academic disciplines. It was for these reasons that approaching women directly became useful.

Direct Approach

Although I eventually managed to access 14 women using the snowball technique, this took a long time, from September 2005 to March 2006, to complete all the interviews. There were moments when I would get completely stuck with no idea about whom to interview next. Some interviewees did not want to lead me to others. When a topic is sensitive, some people may feel uncomfortable about suggesting names of people to be interviewed. The deputy human resources manager of Holy Ghost University, for example, told me that if she directed me to others, they might suspect that she had disclosed details about their health status, because she knew a lot about the personal lives of staff given the nature of her work. Even after I assured her that I would not disclose her role, she seemed uncomfortable and I respected her position and professional ethics.

Approaching total strangers became an option that was quite helpful. I recall the first day I visited Holy Ghost University I had planned to look for the woman whom I had met at a gender conference a few months prior to the fieldwork. On reaching the campus, I was told she was out that day. I asked the secretary if there was another woman lecturer in that department who was on campus. She told me there was one who would be out of class in a few minutes if I could wait. When the lecturer came out, I introduced myself as a lecturer doing research in Holy Ghost. She became interested and took me to her office. I explained my research project to her and asked her if she wished to be interviewed. She accepted but commented: "I do not think there is a problem as one can only say what they feel comfortable to talk about". This was interesting for me with regard to agency of research participants and the need for the researcher to use triangulation for improved reliability of the data collected.

From this research, I learnt that research participants are not just powerless people waiting to be bombarded with any kind of questions. They choose how they will respond and what they will respond to. This view is shared by Thapar-Bjorkert and Henry (2004) when they write about their field experiences with women in India. They note: "Our own experiences in the field show that respondents (and many others who participate in the research process) do exercise power, which not only affects the experience of research, but critically transforms the final product" (p. 365). Reliability and validity of the data are discussed in a later section of this chapter.

I used the direct approach to access all the four men representing management. This method was especially useful to access the Vice Chancellor of Weruini University where I had to employ my negotiating skills to persuade his secretary to explain to him about my research project (see also Chapter Four).

Profile of Research Participants

After a careful selection of the participants described above, I ended up with participants with a set of characteristics, which are summarised in Tables 1 and 2. All the respondents except one were Christians. They were drawn from different ethnic groups in Kenya, which included Kikuyu, Kisii, Luyhia, Luo, Meru, Kamba and Kalenjin.

Out of the 25 men and women I interviewed in this study, 19 were married (all the men were married). Two women were divorced and one woman separated, while the remaining three women were single and had never married. One of the divorced women, Dr. Kaiga (this is a pseudonym as all names have been changed) told me that her status had been a source of ridicule from both men and women. She said that divorce had not been an easy option to take, but she had decided she was better off divorced than being in a failed marriage. The woman who was separated (Prof. Atieno) told me that I was the first person outside her circle of closest friends and family that she had told about it. None of her colleagues knew about it because she thought they might not understand her reason for opting for separation. This confirms the discussion in Chapter Two, that marriage is held with very high regard in Kenya. I felt greatly honoured that these women could open up to me although this was our first meeting. This research made some women able to talk about private issues that they may have found difficult to talk about in another setting. In Chapter Four, the therapeutic nature of research interviews is discussed further.

As indicated in Table 1, the participants represented various positions in their universities, including full professors, lecturers, chaplain, counsellor, librarian and the human resource officer. There were two deans (Prof. Nyaboke and Dr. Kivuu) and three heads of departments (Dr. Wangare, Prof. Atieno and Dr. Atoti). The ages of the respondents ranged from 34 to 60 years.

I had decided from the onset to try and get a representation of women from different age groups, ethnicity, marital status

Table 1: Profile of women participants

Name	University	Position	Marital status	Age	Ethnic group
1. Prof. Atieno	Weruini	Associate Professor	Separated	46	Luo
2. Prof Nyaboke	Weruini	Associate Professor	Married	48	Kisii
3. Dr. Atoti	Weruini	Senior Lecturer	Married	48	Luo
4. Dr. Kaiga	Weruini	Senior Lecturer	Divorced	40	Kikuyu
5. Dr. Wangare	Weruini	Senior Lecturer	Divorced	47	Kikuyu
6. Dr. Muasia	Weruini	Senior Lecturer	Married	54	Kamba
7. Dr. Nkirote	Weruini	Senior Lecturer	Married	55	Meru
8. Mrs Bihanya	Weruini	Lecturer	Married	44	Luyhia
9. Dr. Gaudencia	Weruini	Lecturer	Married	40	Luo
10. Mrs Musoga	Weruini	Lecturer	Married	40	Kikuyu
11. Mrs Munyi	Weruini	Lecturer	Married	40	Kalenjin
12. Mrs Bahati	Holy Ghost	Lecturer	Married	36	Kikuyu
13. Rev. Kibaata	Holy Ghost	Chaplain	Married	37	Meru
14. Mrs Kibet	Holy Ghost	Counsellor	Married	38	Kalenjin
15. Ms Mugasia	Holy Ghost	Lecturer	Single	35	Luyhia
16. Mrs Mwithaga	Holy Ghost	Librarian	Married	45	Kikuyu
17. Ms Mueni	Holy Ghost	Lecturer	Single	37	Kamba
18. Ms Karabo	Holy Ghost	Lecturer & HoD	Single	42	Kisii
19. Mrs Wakaba	Holy Ghost	Lecturer	Married	60	Kikuyu
20. Mrs Wandera	Holy Ghost	Lecturer	Married	56	Luyhia

Table 2: Participants from management

Name	University	Position	Marital status
1. Dr Oduor	Weruini	Director (ACU)	Married
2. Prof Atwoli	Weruini	Board member ACU	Married
3. Prof. Awuondo	Weruini	Vice Chancellor	Married
4. Mrs Mwala	Holy Ghost	Deputy HRM	Married
5. Dr. Kivuu	Holy Ghost	Dean and Ag. Director ACU	Married

and positions in the university to establish if these factors made a difference to the women's experiences. This was not an issue with those in management, as I was not looking at their personal experiences with HIV and AIDS. Other details of the participants are given in the data chapters whenever I use extracts from the interviews. I have avoided too many details that could make it easy for readers especially, in Kenya, to recognise the participants.

Methods Used for Data Collection

I used qualitative methods, which Mason (2002) describes as 'highly exciting' because qualitative methods are concerned with those aspects of life "that matter and in ways that matter" (p. 1). Qualitative research allows the researcher to go into the depth of participants' experiences, social processes and discourses, by using approaches and methodologies that appreciate the depth and richness of data (Mason, 2002). Mason further notes that qualitative research:

> Has an unrivalled capacity to constitute compelling arguments about how things work in particular contexts, ... qualitative research is also 'capable of producing well founded cross-contextual generalities, rather than aspiring to more flimsy de-contextualised versions' (p. 1, emphasis hers).

Qualitative methods were most suitable for the feminist epistemology and ontology of my study. The distinct characteristic of qualitative methods according to Gillham (2000a; 2000b) is that they focus primarily on the stories that people give the researcher, and from these stories issues can be illuminated and help to develop explanations about a certain phenomenon. Gillham (2000a; 2000b) further appreciates the strength of qualitative research in helping the researcher to explore complexities that may be beyond the scope of more controlled approaches.

Further, Campbell (2003) notes that most research on HIV and AIDS has continued to rely on quantitative survey methodologies, which, despite having provided vital information, often contribute little to deeper understanding of the programmes. It has also been argued that in the area of HIV and AIDS, qualitative data provides useful information about the socially constructed experiences that this epidemic presents (Commonwealth Secretariat, 2002). In the next sections, I discuss the actual qualitative methods that I used in this study.

In-depth Conversational Interviews

In this study, I adopted what I refer to as 'in-depth and conversational interviews.' Blackmore (1999) writes about using conversational interviews in her research where the storytelling genre of the interview could be adjusted to have a more informal discussion taking the form of a conversation.

On the use of conversational interviews, Merrill (1999) observes that:

> The interview dialogue becomes a more equal two way process as the interviewer and the interviewee interact in a conversation and it is not only the interviewer who asks questions. Rather, the interviewer should be prepared to share life experiences with the interviewees (p. 59).

Like Merrill, I wanted to make use of conversations in order to have a two-way dialogue with my interviewees. I understood conversational interviews to be a process where the research participants and I would be engaged in dialogue. The participants could ask me questions and I was prepared to respond to them. I felt morally obliged to talk about my life as they too were talking about theirs (see also Chapter Four). I carried out this study from an ontological position, which suggests that people's knowledge, views, understanding and interpretations are meaningful for the generation of knowledge. Put differently, the participants' views and opinions have helped to bring to light issues that would not be apparent in more closed and structured methods of data collection (Burke, 2002; Campbell, 2003; Holstein and Gubrium, 1995;Mason, 2002).

By use of conversational interviewing, I had the advantage of being able to have a collaborative dialogue with my women participants. I could respond to their questions and ask for clarifications too as noted by other researchers (Acker et al., 1991; Blackmore, 1999; Burke, 2002; Mason, 2002; Merrill, 1999). This was also in recognition of the freedom of choice of the interviewees and I as we all had different reactions to the interview (Griffiths, 1998; Holstein and Gubrium, 1995). I used what Oakley (1990; 1992) refers to as non-hierarchical interview where reciprocity is allowed, the interviewee can ask questions and the interviewer too invests their own personal identity. I was, however, careful not to turn the interviewing sessions into therapeutic encounters (Mason, 2002), which is not the aim of a research interview.

Nonetheless, it is important to note that there are researchers who have found the therapeutic nature of interviews to be an advantage to the participants, an issue I discuss further in the following chapter. In a research interview, participants can reflect on their experiences as they are offered an opportunity to talk about themselves and the situation they are in (Burgess, 1988; Opie, 1992). For some women, this research interview may be the only chance they find to have someone interested in their experiences (see Chapter Four). This is one way interviews can become empowering encounters rather than be exploitative, depending on the power relationships (Opie, 1992).

While I adopted a conversational tone, the interviews were guided by some broad topics or guiding themes (Blackmore, 1999). These themes helped to create an atmosphere that was conducive for the women to talk about their experiences in a safe conversational mode (Appleby, 1994; Burgess, 1982, 1988; Burke, 2002; Mason, 2002; Mauthner and Doucet, 1998). Likewise, Yin (2003) notes that although case study interviews should be as open-ended as possible, a bit of a structure or guiding themes help to keep the consistency of the issue under inquiry. The guiding themes helped to keep the interviews on track because some women could talk about issues that were unrelated to the study, but I was able to bring them back to the main topics. In Appendix 6, I have provided the guide that I followed during the conversational interviews and the elite interviews. However, in some of the interviews, I did not manage to follow the schedule due to varying circumstances, which I discuss in Chapter Four.

From past experiences with interviewing, I learnt that it was better to leave the interview to run like a normal conversation without following too many rules and guidelines that could make it lose the natural aspects of real life research. On this, Burgess (1988) notes that it is important that interview conversations remain focused to the issues being studied. This means that the conversation needs to be guided by the researcher (Appleby, 1994). As the researcher, I had already read sufficiently around the topic of the research, hence would have been unfair to expect the interviewees to be able to grasp the issues without some explanations and guiding (Hollway and Jefferson, 2000). I played this role of explaining and guiding as I have detailed in Appendices 6 and 7.

Besides the conversational interviews, I also carried out some focused interviews with five persons representing the management of the two universities.

Focused Interviews with Management

The second set of interviews fell under what Yin (2003) and Gillham (2000a: 63; 2000b: 81-83) refer to as the 'focused' and 'elite' interviews respectively. These are usually shorter than the in-depth interviews described above. The focused interview is preferred when dealing with senior people because it is short and focuses on straight and open questions. The guiding questions I used in these interviews are in Appendix 7.

My purpose in using this type of interview was to benefit from its advantages when interviewing senior people; focused interviews give interviewees a chance to be in control of the interview "as they may not submit to being tamely 'interviewed' where you direct a series of questions at them" (Gillham, 2000b: 82). Focused interviews are also more "likely to have a particularly comprehensive grasp of the wider context and to be privy to information that is withheld from others. Quite simply, their perspective is different" (Gillham, 2000b: 81).

Focused interviews can also be beneficial in providing the researcher with ideas on where and how to collect further data. For example, they can, among other benefits, provide information on where and what kind of documents and records one can find, permission to gain access to them, contacts of more relevant people to be interviewed that could emerge in the interview. True to this quality of focused interviews, it was through some of them that I was able to get a good grasp of what was happening in the universities. Two of the interviewees (Prof Atwoli and Dr. Oduor) were helpful in directing me to places where I could get further information. Before I describe the other methods of data collection I used in this study, I briefly discuss the issue of tape recording of these interviews.

Tape-recording of Interviews

Every researcher has to make a decision on how to keep a record of the interviews in an accurate and ethical manner. Reiss (2000), for example, says that he decided not to tape-record his interviews but to take notes because of his own experiences of being tape-recorded in an interview where he was unable to make any off-the-cuff remarks. While there are disadvantages in relying on memory to take notes after the interview, Reiss (2000) notes that he chose to take notes so as not to put his interviewees through the same discomfort he had experienced as an interviewee.

My own experience with interviewing, for example, during my other research with university staff (Kamau, 2001) showed that interviewees could become uncomfortable with tape-recording. They tended to talk more when the tape was off. Some of my interviewees in the earlier research commented that they would rather talk 'off the record' although they had been assured of anonymity. Indeed some researchers have argued that tape recording can inhibit free expression. Preece and Ntseane (2004), for example, write about their focus groups on HIV and AIDS intervention strategies in Botswana, where they decided against tape-recording to allow more natural discussions.

Nevertheless, my experience during the pilot study of this research, in which I used both tape-recording and note taking made me decide to tape-record all interviews. Taking notes caused an interruption to the flow of our conversations and I ended up not writing everything as I did with the recorded ones. On note-taking during interviews, Wengraf (2001) comments that it breaks the contact and rapport with the interviewee and it interferes with the flow of information. In addition, Gillham (2000b) argues that many interviewees tend to forget that they are being recorded once the interview is in full flow and yet, taking notes can be continuously inhibiting to the flow of the interview. Where the interviews are short, taking notes can be adequate but this may not work well with longer interviews, as was the case in this study, unlike the earlier one I mention above.

Furthermore, listening to the recorded interviews also helps to recapture the scene all over again, the tone of voice and the expressions, which would be completely lost if not recorded. When negotiating for access and consent with my potential interviewees, I explained that I would tape-record the interviews and gave an assurance that I would make anonymous any details that could be used to identify them. By changing all the names of the interviewees and by providing only basic information about the case universities, I hope I have managed to protect the actual identities of my respondents. The details I have provided in Tables 1 and 2 can fit many people working in universities because I did not give any characteristics that would be unique to the participants. There are also many universities in Kenya fitting the characteristics I have provided for Weruini and Holy Ghost. Two of my university colleagues who read my work were unable to identify these universities.

To make the recording less intimidating, I used a tiny digital recorder which, however, created a lot of interest amongst many of my interviewees, who being researchers themselves, found it user-friendly and wanted to know how they could acquire it. This interest on the recorder seemed to have helped to ease any tension that could have been associated with recording, although none of the interviewees told me that they minded being taped. However, one interviewee seemed not to have consented to the interview because she did not talk much during the interview but opened up more after the interview. It was difficult for me to establish if the problem was due to the tape-recording, or whether she was not comfortable with the topic, or if it was another manifestation of the silences that this study sought to establish. This case is discussed further in Chapter Four where I address the ethical challenges of negotiating access and consent. Apart from interviews, I also made use of my field notes and the AIDS policy of Weruini University.

Field notes

My field notes constituted part of the data collection. The field notes or research diary written by the researcher can be said to be a counterpart of the information given by other research participants (Bell, 1998). On field notes, Bell asks: "shouldn't the researcher also be 'called to account' for his or her own experiences, in the same way as informants are asked to be?" (1998: 82).

I decided to use my own observations about the field process as part of my data. My diary notes included my observations, field activities and thoughts, as I encountered different experiences in the course of data collection. In the process of data analysis, I found my field notes useful as they helped clarify some of the data. These notes and reflections also helped me to put the interview texts into context. It is from these notes that I kept a record of some of my observations, reflections and thoughts on certain issues like power relations, consent and disclosure, which are discussed in Chapter Four. Unlike Bell (1998) who notes that she did not record her own private thoughts and anxieties in her field notes, I recorded my own private feelings of the process of data collection.

I carried out this study from an ontological perspective that saw interactions, actions and behaviour as central in helping me to understand ways in which the selected universities were responding to HIV and AIDS in relation to the senior women staff. The observations recorded in the field notes helped me to understand what was happening in the two universities from more than one angle. For a clearer understanding of how the universities were responding to HIV and AIDS, it was necessary that I went beyond the information provided in interviews. I found my diary notes helpful in prompting me into new sites for data collection as I discovered issues that I had not thought about before going into the field (Brown and Dowling, 1998).

My field notes became part of my data collection and making sense of these notes remained part of my data analysis, a fact noted by several researchers (Brown and Dowling, 1998; Burke, 2002; Kvale, 1996; Moyles, 2002; Nias et al., 1989; Smit, 2006; Williams, 1990). On use of such notes throughout the research process, Kvale (1996) notes:

> It may be worthwhile for the interviewer to set aside 10 minutes of quiet time after each interview to recall and reflect on what has been learned from the particular interview, including the interpersonal interaction. These immediate impressions, based on the interviewer's empathetic access to the meanings communicated, may – in the form of

notes or simply recorded onto the interview tape – provide a valuable context for the later analysis of transcripts (p. 129).

Chapter Four is based on my impressions from the interviews and the entire fieldwork, which I recorded in my diary. This chapter is, for me, another way of bringing to the open, issues of research that rarely find space in the written text. It was another way that this study unearths silences especially related to areas of research that are hardly talked or written about. Field notes therefore played an important role in helping me to keep in touch with all aspects of my research.

The other source of data that is used in this research is the AIDS policy of Weruini University. At the time of my research, Holy Ghost University did not have an AIDS policy.

Documentary Evidence

As is characteristic of case studies, it is crucial that one makes use of multiple methods to increase the chances of understanding the case in greater detail, to get multiple layers of data for more depth and indeed discover new insights on the situation (Mason, 2002; Robson, 2002; Yin, 2003). I used AIDS policy of Weruini University to gain a clear understanding of the institutional responses to HIV and AIDS.

I used Weruini AIDS policy as data to show what the university had put as their commitment to the epidemic (Chapter Eight). This public document is then compared with what the women said in the conversational interviews, with an aim of establishing whether the official position recognised the private challenges of senior women staff.

Reliability and Validity of the Methodology

Concerning questions of reliability and validity of this study, I followed the ideas of Bassey (1999: 74-77). Reliability is defined as "the extent to which, research findings can be repeated, given the same circumstances" (ibid. p. 75). Bassey (1999) defines validity "as the extent to which a research fact or finding is what it is claimed to be" (1999 p. 75). Since my study was not necessarily of a 'theory-seeking' type, but rather of a 'story-telling' type (hence not involving direct cause and effect), I adapted what Lincoln and Guba (1985) refer to as trustworthiness of the data (cited in Bassey, 1999). Bassey (ibid.) develops this concept of trustworthiness further by raising the following questions that case study researchers should reflect on if their work is to be termed as trustworthy or reliable:

- Has there been prolonged engagement with data sources?

- Has there been prolonged observation of emerging issues?

- Have raw data been adequately checked with their sources?

- Has a critical friend thoroughly tried to challenge the findings?

- Does the case record provide an adequate audit trail?

I will now look at some of these questions, which I find relevant to my study. All the questions are taken directly from Bassey (1999: 76-77).

Has there been prolonged engagement with data sources?

Bassey (1999:76-77) defines prolonged engagement as spending enough time with the case to become fully immersed in its issues, while also building the trust of the research participants and avoiding misleading information. I spent adequate time in the two universities because the whole fieldwork took a total of seven months to complete (September 2004 to March 2005). During this time, I visited these institutions not less than three times every week. I got involved in informal discussions with many different people in the institutions.

While observation was not a formal method of data collection, I could not avoid noticing what was going on, since I was in the institutions. Sometimes when I had to wait for people to interview, I would get a chance to read through university newsletters that provided me with information on what was going on in the campus. I noted any important observations in my research diary. For example, I noted that in the seven months that I was in the two institutions, there was nothing in their newsletters that was specifically about HIV and AIDS. These notes, as I have noted elsewhere in this chapter, were also helpful in clarifying some issues that came up in the interviews.

Has there been prolonged observation of emerging issues?

During the seven months of data collection, I was able to make observations and take field notes, which were useful in giving me a clear picture of the issues I was studying. I had gone to the field with the assumption that the universities were focusing more on students in their responses to HIV and AIDS. I was able to confirm this by visiting various students' activities: for example, at Holy Ghost University there was a mobile voluntary counselling and testing clinic (VCT) for two weeks during the month of November 2004, and I was able to talk with the counsellor working there. I learnt that the VCT had been organised by the students and that no staff member visited it in the two weeks. I also visited the 'I Choose Life' (ICL) offices of both universities and got an impression of the activities that students were involved in. ICL is an international NGO with a leading behaviour-change peer-education programme targeting HIV and AIDS in Kenyan universities. It was started in 2002 and it had established programmes in seven universities across Kenya at the time of this study (this was derived from my field notes).

I also recorded in my field notes a conversation I had with a medical doctor working at the Holy Ghost clinic. I generally wanted to know if the clinic was dealing with staff issues related to HIV and AIDS. The doctor told me that since the clinic was small, mainly offering first aid services, it was difficult to establish patients' underlying health problems. Serious health issues were referred to the big hospitals. On being asked about the problem of HIV and AIDS at Holy Ghost and in the country in general, he said that he saw lack of connection between clinical work and AIDS prevention and support work. He noted that doctors just receive patients in hospitals, assess them and prescribe drugs without any more follow-up.

Through all these conversations and my observations I was able to have a thorough search of all the salient features I needed for my study and focus on those that I thought were helpful in answering my research question.

Have raw data been adequately checked with their sources?

According to Bassey (1999) and others, such as Wengraf (2001), it is good practice to take the transcribed interview back to the interviewees to check that the report is an accurate record of what they said and to confirm that they are still willing to have the information used in the research. This is important for the trustworthiness of the data especially in cases where more than one interview is required from each participant (Onsongo, 2005). However, this is one area where I made a conscious decision not to take back the transcripts to the interviewees unless they requested them. Only one woman requested that I give her the transcribed text, as she wanted a record of what we had talked about for her future use.

I reflected a great deal on the ethics of my decisions. First, I had decided that one interview per person would be enough because the issues I was covering were easily exhausted in one interview. Also, the conversational and open nature of the interviews made it easy for us to cover almost all that I required for the research. I also had a chance to talk at length with many women after the formal interviews were over (see Chapter Four). This gave me the opportunity to clarify issues that may not have been clear, which I recorded in my diary. I, therefore, did not see the need for a second interview and as Merrill (1999) argues, it is most essential to check with interviewees where multiple interviews are involved.

In addition, given my reflections on the ethics of a sensitive study like this one, which I address fully in Chapter Four, I decided that taking transcripts back to the interviewees could act as a reminder of private and sensitive issues they had disclosed, with no plan of having to see them printed on paper. I thought it was more ethical not to return transcripts to them as it may have rekindled the painful memories that were talked about in the interviews.

As I discuss in the next question, I also discussed this dilemma with one of my feminist friends who had just completed her doctoral research, which also targeted senior academics in Kenya. In her case she returned the transcripts and she said she had occasions when the women changed almost everything she had recorded, especially issues that concerned the private domain. Based on her experiences, she advised me not to return transcripts, especially in a sensitive study that also involved participants who were more powerful than the researcher, as was the case with both our studies (see Onsongo, 2005).

Has a critical friend thoroughly tried to challenge the findings?

I have two women friends who were also carrying out feminist research in Kenyan universities during the period I did mine. These women offered me useful peer debriefing. We started meeting from the beginning of the study and I would keep them up-to-date about how my data collection process was progressing. I tested my interview schedule with both of them. They continued to offer useful feedback. Since these women were my peers, they were generous with their time and we developed a relationship based on honesty and humility. Hence, they could give me critical feedback without damaging our friendship. I have also offered similar feedback to their work.

Three independent readers also read the work and they too provided some critical feedback that I were incorporated in the final report of the study. In addition, I presented part of the research findings at two conferences, namely 'The 6th Pan-African Social

Work Conference held in April, 2005, and the CHE and UNESCO Workshop on 'Mainstreaming HIV and AIDS in Institutions of Higher Learning in Kenya' held in November 2005. It was at this conference where I finally met my mentor Prof. Michael Kelly and we had a chance for a face-to-face discussion on the progress of my work and he gave some very useful feedback. I also made a presentation in an official launch of an AIDS Control Unit in one of the Kenyan universities held on 8th March 2006. Many members of Kenya's academia attended these occasions. From their reactions, I was able to look at my data again and reflect on my interpretations. It was in the CHE and UNESCO conferences where I became aware of the challenges that I may face in disseminating findings of a sensitive study like this one (see Chapter Four).

Does the case record provide an adequate audit trail?

I have kept all the field notes and the interviews (both recorded and transcribed versions). I have included one conversational interview in Appendix 8. Another important feature in reaching the conclusions of a trustworthy case study is to provide a sound explanation of how the data has been analysed, which I discuss next.

Data Analysis

Data analysis includes data management, which is a long process that begins right at the first steps of designing the research question and continues to the end of the research report. From the beginning of this research project, I made several analytical decisions which include the following: the literature I have reviewed, my choice of theories that have guided the study, my methodology, the questions to asked, and whom to ask. All these decisions became part of my data analysis.

While in the field collecting data, I continued making some analysis through summarising, coding, filing, and observing patterns and themes that guided the rest of the data collection. The data collection exercise took place from September 2004 to March 2005. I had initially expected that the whole exercise of data collection would take only three months. However, I found out that this was not practical as there were periods when I could not manage to access people to interview because many of them were busy. The ACU director of Weruini University was out of the country from September to December 2004, for example, and his schedule was tight as he had many pending issues when he returned. It was not an easy to get hold of such people for interviews.

There were periods within the seven months when I had no interviews and was not visiting the universities. I decided to spend my 'free time' listening to the recorded interviews. I listened to each of the interviews twice before I started transcribing them. I wanted to be sure that I was hearing what the interviewees actually said, while also listening to my own voice in the interviews.

There were moments when I needed to take breaks between the recording and the second listening just to be sure that I was hearing the voices clearly. Before making any deeper analysis of data, I wanted to be sure that I got the real meanings behind the words said and my own notes. I ended up with about 120 pages of text from the interviews and 35 pages of field notes. This was an enormous amount of data that required careful handling if I was to remain faithful to the voices of the research participants (see also Chapter Seven).

Having typed out the interviews, I moved away from listening to reading so that I could start doing some coding. However, before doing any coding, I read through the texts a few times to be sure that my own attitudes, values and perspectives were not taking precedence over what the interviewees said. I have remained conscious of the fact that it is not enough to give people a voice by interviewing them; it is equally important that their voices are not 'erased' by turning away from their words (hooks, 1994), which can easily happen if the listening to the interviewees' voices during the analysis is not thorough and sensitive.

With the large volume of data at hand, I decided analyse it using the computer software known as Nvivo, which is used for qualitative data analysis. The use of Nvivo was helpful in data management, but before exporting the files from MS Word to Nvivo, I did some initial coding of some of the themes that were emerging. This initial coding made the searching for codes/nodes in Nvivo much easier. Using the software, I created a total of 40 free nodes (of some of the recurring themes which I had coded in MS Word). Some of the codes that emerged included the following: silence, stigma, sexuality, care, support, challenges facing women in the two universities, doctorates and women's careers, balancing personal and professional roles, and university responses to HIV and AIDS.

Having formulated the codes, I then performed electronic searches using Nvivo, which was just like cutting and pasting. I carried out several of these searches and made coding reports, which I exported back to MS Word. These are the files I worked with to pull out extracts, which I found relevant for different themes addressed in each of the chapters. The chapter headings have emerged from the themes pulled out from the data.

From the themes, I looked for the plausibility of the data. This involved asking myself questions like: did the themes, trends and patterns make sense? How valid and reliable were they? I did this by looking for intervening patterns, and issues and concepts in the literature that could help explain these patterns, concepts, issues and themes. I kept asking myself, what did the data as a whole mean beyond the particular men and women I had interviewed (Brown and Dowling, 1998).

Using evidence from literature and other studies, I have been able to argue that the findings of this study could be seen as instances of structural and policy issues in universities. These issues are not unique to the women I interviewed. The literature helped me to understand that the issues that arose from the interviews could be raised beyond the people interviewed.

In the data analysis, I continued to think about how the initial questions and data related to the final product which resulted in this book. Additionally, I continued to be aware and reflexive of the changes I, too, underwent from the start of the project to the end, as this continuously influenced how I interpreted and understood the data. Some questions that would come to mind during the analysis included the following: what was it in my own talk and questioning that contributed to the responses of the interviewees? How could I read their reflexivity in their responses? Did the interviews help the respondents to reflect on the issues under study in ways that could contribute to change at personal and probably at institutional level?

Throughout the data analysis, I continued to have discussions with professional colleagues, my supervisor, other tutors, students and further review of literature. All these ideas and interpretations assisted me in making more sense of the issues arising from the data. However, the final decisions on what has been written were entirely my own. On this, Burke (2002) notes that her data analysis was shared with different people and in different situations, some of them planned while others occurred spontaneously through conversations.

Summary and Conclusion

Writing this chapter after completing my fieldwork makes me realise that research designs, which appear in advance to effectively translate theoretical questions into a workable formula for empirical investigations, do not always work out in practice. Some unexpected events (some of which can be discovered during the pilot study) may require adjustments. These include the realisation that what appeared initially feasible is impractical or does not take into account newly emerging factors that are of importance.

In this chapter, I have laid out the processes that I followed in the data collection exercise, including a theoretical basis for each of the choices made. I have also shown some areas where a few adjustments were required after I was faced with realities in the field. Having incorporated these realities, I was able to come up with a design that helped me to address my research questions in the best way possible.

Nonetheless, this being a sensitive study, I was faced with a number of ethical challenges, many of which I had not envisaged. In my literature search, I did not find much written about the challenges of researching a sensitive topic. For this reason, I decided to set aside the next chapter for ethical issues.

= 4 ════════════════════════════

Researching a Sensitive Topic:
Ethical Issues and Other Challenges*

Introduction

Research on a sensitive topic like HIV and AIDS confronts researchers with many difficult ethical questions. Ethical issues in research are concerned with rights and welfare of all those included in a study.

In this chapter I discuss the ethical challenges that I faced while studying a sensitive topic. I begin the chapter by discussing my understanding of ethics, while also explaining why my study qualified to be termed 'sensitive'. I then move on to discuss and explain the various ethical challenges and dilemmas that I was faced with during various stages and aspects of my data collection, analysis and dissemination.

I include this chapter in my thesis because I did not find much literature about the ethics of researching a sensitive topic. I felt this was an area where researchers had chosen to be silent about their private experiences in the field. Silence is a major and recurring theme in this thesis. Therefore, I decided not to be 'silent' about my experiences in the field that would be seen to lie in the 'private' and 'personal' aspects of the study.

---

* A revised version of this chapter has since been published with Prof. Onsongo as a journal article - Onsongo, J. and Kamau, N. (2009). "Researching Academics in Kenyan Universities: A Reflection on Research Ethics," *Journal of Sociology and Education in Africa*. Special Edition, Vol. 8, No. 2 (2009): 187-214.

Ethics and Research

A World Council of Churches study document on AIDS (WCC, 1997) describes ethics as a theory that:

> ...clarifies questions about right and wrong, but also demonstrates their complexity: most ethical theories, and many moral judgements are contestable...Nevertheless, meaningful and constructive frameworks developed by ethical reflections over the ages can be used to examine the facts and values in question, leading to a degree of consensus, or at least a mutual understanding of divergent views (p. 50).

The above description of ethics shows that ethical theories are based on differing views, values and principles. I decided that my ethical decisions would be guided by the British Educational Research Association ethical guidelines (BERA, 2004) and feminist principles of doing ethical research. I also considered the values and beliefs of my research participants bearing in mind the sensitive nature of the topic of my research.

In Chapter Three, I have discussed feminist methodology that guided my research. Feminist methodology "implies a connection between politics, ethics and epistemology" (Ramazanoglu and Holland, 2002:102). Ethical considerations make the feminist researcher accountable for the knowledge they may produce and since feminist research is about fairness, respect, and promoting the good of others, ethics become central.

The complexities of researching people's private lives and then bringing these accounts into the public, which form an integral part of feminist research, raise ethical issues for the researcher that need to be expressed throughout the research and writing up process (Mauthner et al., 2002). This chapter plays the role of expressing the ethical challenges that I faced throughout the research process.

The Sensitive Nature of this Study

A study focusing on university women's experiences with HIV and AIDS is, indeed, sensitive. This is because HIV and AIDS is surrounded by silence, ignorance, secrecy, stigma and discrimination (Kelly, 2001; Nzioka, 2000). In addition, many educated and well-off Africans do not want to identify themselves with a problem that for a long time has been associated with low class, sexually irresponsible people (Barnett and Whiteside, 2002; Campbell, 2003; Ochola-Ayayo, 1997; Shisanya, 2002; Wood, 2002).

Lee and Renzetti (1993) note that a piece of research is considered sensitive not only because of the topic, but also the social context in which it occurs. From the beginning of the data collection, I was aware that this study could be the subject of controversy (Shahidian, 2001). I knew that the interviews would touch a chord in people's private lives in ways that could be stressful if revealed. Nonetheless, I felt that this study was justified in Kenya, which continues to be devastated by the AIDS pandemic (NACC, 2003; PWC, 2004; Udoto, 2004).

The situation of the pandemic in higher education is equally devastating, requiring urgent attention (Nyutho et al., 2005; Owino, 2004). In the report of an East African regional conference on developing policies and practices for mainstreaming HIV and AIDS in institutions of higher learning, it is stated that:

> Despite the fact that various indicators show considerable HIV and AIDS impact on institutions of higher learning, responses to the pandemic by the institutions leave a lot to be desired... where integration has been done, it has largely been in the domain of health or medical faculties. HIV and AIDS demands a coordinated response from every institution of higher learning (CHE and UNESCO, 2004: vii)

As the above quotation indicates, there is some urgency for interventions that would go beyond health and medical interventions. I considered that a study that would take into consideration the experiences of senior university women with this pandemic was timely. My readings of other feminist research helped me in arguing that even sensitive and private experiences need to be studied as they help to discern and uncover actual facts of people's lives and experiences (Doucet and Mauthner, 2002; Mauthner, 2000; Mauthner and Doucet, 1998; Oakley, 1992). Many such experiences, especially by women, "have been hidden, inaccessible, suppressed, distorted, misunderstood and ignored" (Du Bois, 1983: 109).

For a clearer understanding of a sensitive topic, I draw on Lee and Renzetti's definition:

> One that potentially poses for those involved, a substantial threat, the emergence of which renders problematic for researcher and/or researched the collection, holding, and/or dissemination of research data (1993: 5) (emphasis in original).

In this research, I asked participants to talk about their experiences with a disease that is surrounded by stigma. The women talked about experiences in their families that they said had been kept secret. Therefore, they were revealing information that could be problematic if their families or even other colleagues knew about it.

Some of the women in one of the universities also said that there was discrimination against those infected, as I discuss in Chapter Eight. I was also enquiring about what the universities had done about HIV and AIDS, an issue that was both problematic and political as I was to learn later on.

Threats that research may pose to individual participants may be broad, ranging from dealing with areas in the individual's lives that are private, stressful or sacred to the implications of what they reveal to their public spaces especially at the workplace. Research into sensitive topics may be seen as involving some potential risk or cost to those being researched (Lee and Renzetti, 1993). As a result, a sensitive study requires serious ethical considerations throughout the research process, from the preparation stage, to data collection, and dissemination of findings (Alderson and Morrow, 2004; Lee, 2001; Shahidian, 2001).

Specifically, I had to ensure that my participants' rights, my methodological requirements and my dissemination responsibilities were addressed satisfactorily (Hays and Murphy, 2003). In order to do this, I reflected on ethical questions that I thought relevant to me as a social researcher. Shahidian (2001) summarises them as:

> Who is the researcher and where does he or she stand in relation to the research topic, how does the researcher define the concepts, choose the tools, and address the various challenges of fieldwork? What are the ethical dimensions of the research? How does the researcher respond to them?' (p. 55)

One of the important ethical decisions I made from the onset was to change all the names of the two universities and respondents. I decided to stick to names rather than numbers or letters as I felt that use of 'real' names made the experiences remain close to the people. I have found research that uses letters or numbers alienating because I cannot see the link between the actual people and the data. I wanted to avoid this in my study where the key objective was to listen to and record women's experiences.

Even though all the names have been changed, I have used names that remind me of the women as much as possible as this has helped to keep these women 'close' to me. I give titles (Ms., Mrs., Dr., or Prof.) to all the women as they introduced themselves to me by their titles. Only one introduced herself to me by her first name only, and I decided to refer to her as such. This was an important ethical decision for me, as I wanted to refer to these women the way I thought they would find most comfortable. The present chapter does not provide any definitive answers to the ethical challenges that a sensitive topic poses to researchers. However, it makes a contribution to this important area of research ethics.

Gaining the Research Participant's Trust

My research participants included senior men and women of the two universities, the Kenyan university community in general, and other people in organisations like the Commission for Higher Education (CHE) and UNESCO that were working directly with universities on the issue of HIV and AIDS.

From the time I designed my research project, I planned to use different ways to gain the confidence of the research participants. This was important so that they could trust my motives for a study of this nature. To achieve this, I attended conferences, workshops and seminars and continued writing articles on gender issues in one of the local daily newspapers (I write opinion articles in the *Daily Nation*, a leading Kenyan newspaper). It was while in some of these forums that I met some of my participants for both the pilot and the main study. Presenting academic papers in these conferences helped to draw people towards me, as they wanted to discuss these presentations further.

Some of the research participants also mentioned that they had read my articles in the newspaper. Shahidian (2001) notes that public exposure helped him to gain trust from his research community:

> ... Increased exposure through the lectures and media coverage facilitated my contact with new people, enhanced my credentials in the community and drew data to me. "This level of exposure", as one female interviewee put it, "not only helped us to understand you, but also to find you too vulnerable to pull something funny up your sleeve" (p. 67).

In dealing with a sensitive topic and context, it is important that potential interviewees understand the researchers' values and ideals. Such an understanding gives them the confidence to talk about their lives. In addition, Kenyan universities are hierarchical, where senior academics and administrators may have little time for junior academics (like I was). In this regard, it was crucial that the participants viewed me as a serious academic hence worth their time (Tang, 2002). In one case, I gained access to a senior male professor by reminding him about a conference in which we both had participated and presented papers in 2001. He agreed to be interviewed and was keen to hear how I was progressing with my academic career since the conference.

Throughout the research period, I continued to attend gatherings where I thought I could meet with my potential participants. In one conference organised by CHE, where all Kenyan universities and teacher training colleges were represented, I was able to meet the director of the ACU at Weruini University. I explained my research to him and he gave me an appointment for an interview. Prior to this conference, I had tried to contact him without success as he had been out of the country for almost three months. Even after he returned, my attempts to get him in his office had failed. Meeting this man in such a forum made him consider me as a colleague and hence his acceptance to be interviewed.

The conference also created an opportunity for me to learn what universities said they were doing about HIV and AIDS without having to talk to people individually. This, therefore, became another method of data gathering that helped to increase the trustworthiness of my research findings (see also Chapter Three).

In addition to gaining entry in the public arena, there was still the challenge of approaching individual participants and negotiating access and consent.

Negotiating Access and Consent

In any kind of research, the values of respect, trust and clear information need to consider issues of access and consent (Alderson and Morrow, 2004). I found access and consent intertwined. I had first to make contact with potential participants before explaining to them the study objective and then seeking their consent to be interviewed.

For the 25 interviews, I applied different techniques of negotiating access and consent, because each case was unique. I mainly used a snowball sampling technique, which is commonly used in situations where accessing potential participants is seen to be challenging (Browne, 2005; Miller, 1998; Robson, 2002; Shahidian, 2001; Standing, 1998; and Tang, 2002). For the management staff, approaching them directly was effective. I also sent four letters; one to the Vice Chancellor and the Deputy Vice Chancellor (DVC) of Holy Ghost and to two DVCs of Weruini, when it became difficult to get these people in their offices.

From the beginning, I knew that gaining access to senior university staff willing to talk about HIV and AIDS, would not be easy. Miller (1998: 63) notes that snowball sampling "is a widely recognised technique in qualitative research concerned with accessing stigmatised groups". Although my participants could not be viewed as stigmatised, the topic of my study was sensitive and stigmatising. It was on this premise that I decided to make use of this method of accessing and seeking women's consent.

In addition, I chose to depend on verbal consent only because, as Miller and Bell (2002: 54) point out, "written consent has implications for those trying to access hidden groups or those who are difficult to access". Indeed it is also applicable where people may not want anything bearing their signatures as evidence that they gave such an interview.

I chose the snowball technique as one way of getting started, although I had learnt in my pilot study that it would not be wise to rely on it entirely. This is because potential participants may have found it difficult to refuse when approached by a person well known to them and in some cases by people more senior than themselves. On this, Alderson and Morrow (2004) observe that consent is influenced by the information given about the research to the participants. They need to evaluate the information given and then decide if they would like to participate.

The problem with the snowball technique is that the link person may choose to give information in a way not intended by the researcher (Shahidian, 2001). This could make people consent without a clear understanding of what they are getting themselves into. In one case, a participant who agreed to provide me with a contact decided to call her on my behalf. She made this call even before I had given her enough information concerning my study (I had just mentioned that it was touching on the issue of HIV and AIDS). We had just met when I mentioned that I would ask her to link me with her colleagues. I heard what she told the other woman. She gave a slightly different version of what my study was about, saying that I was interviewing people who were conversant with the university policies on HIV and AIDS. This information obscured the fact that I needed more personal experiences from the women participants. The woman agreed to give me an appointment. During the interview, I was able to explain the objective of my study to her. I also clarified that I was also interested in her personal experiences with HIV and AIDS in addition to her views on what the university was doing about the pandemic. She was comfortable with this explanation and we had a rich conversation.

From this experience, I learnt that consent is something that has to be continuously reassessed and renegotiated. I realised that noting down challenges like that in my research diary became an ethics checklist to which I could refer to as the research progressed (Miller and Bell, 2002). One cannot claim to be fully prepared at the onset of the fieldwork. However, I had prepared some ethical guidelines before starting the main research which I updated regularly as the research progressed (see Appendix 2).

In another case, one of my participants, at my request, contacted her female colleague on my behalf and went ahead to set an appointment (I call this woman Dr. Muasia). Although I was given her telephone number, my attempts to contact her before the interview date were not successful. Even though I still briefed Dr. Muasia on the objective of my study just before we started the interview, she seemed rather secretive and did not talk much throughout the session. This however changed at the end of the interview when I gave her a chance to ask me a question.

I gave each participant the opportunity to ask a question at the end of the interview. I found this useful in a sensitive topic where people may take more time to feel comfortable but may relax when allowed to ask a question. These questions elicited additional information and helped to clarify issues not explored earlier (Gillham, 2000b).

The question Dr. Muasia asked after the interview was why I was concerned with HIV and AIDS in the university. I explained to her more or less as I had done before the interview. It seemed she had not paid attention to my explanation at the beginning because she began to talk more after this. Unfortunately, she had to leave for another meeting, but she was starting to communicate more deeply. This continued in the car when I gave her a lift to her meeting. Here she was much more open and relaxed than during the recorded interview. On further discussion in the car, she confirmed that she had accepted to be interviewed because she had a special interest in HIV and AIDS (field notes, November 16, 2004). This was surprising because she had not shown much interest in the subject during the interview.

The dilemma for me was that the discussion in the car was off the record and I knew it would be ethically wrong to use that as data. This is because, she too was aware that the research context was over. I made an ethical decision that any verbatim quotation of the interviewees would only be from the recorded interviews (It is for this reason that Dr. Muasia's interview is not used when I discuss the findings of this study). However, I have used some information that I noted in my research diary but not in verbatim form. I use my field notes only where I found they were important for me to illustrate another issue raised in the interviews.

I did not get the opportunity to confirm the reason for Dr. Muasia's attitude. My guess was that she either had a misconception about my study, or she simply felt uncomfortable with the issues raised in the interview. She may also have gained confidence, and, indeed developed more trust, at the end of the interview (Brannen, 1988). Alternatively, this woman may have consented simply because a friend had requested her to. Since I had promised it was a one meeting interview, I did not request her for a second one. Instead, I took it as a learning experience (Miller and Bell, 2002). She may also have been silenced by the fact that the interview was held in her office. She left the door open and students kept coming in and out. I hoped she would lock the office but she did not, yet I had no control over the context (see another section in the present chapter on interview context).

Related to the question about whether participants have fully consented or not, Alderson and Morrow (2004) point out that:

> People may, however, be afraid, or too embarrassed, to say no unless they are given a respectful chance to refuse, withdraw, or agree to take part in some or all parts of the research' (p. 97).

In my case, I think Dr. Muasia found it difficult to turn me away, especially because we happened to have a common friend. The fact that we were both academics and expected to assist each other in research – a point that has also been raised by Tang (2002) – might also have contributed to her feeling obliged to carry on with the interview. I could not have known her attitude unless she told me and given that she was a much more senior person to me both in age and in academic position, I did not envisage this problem until I noticed she was not quite willing to talk. However, this could in itself be a reflection of the silencing nature of the topic under study. I decided to have a much shorter interview with her, focusing on general issues rather than the personal ones I discussed with other participants. This way, I hope, I did not appear to be intruding in her life.

If faced with such a situation, Alderson and Morrow (2004) advise that:

> ...it is respectful to talk for a while and then end the interview positively and thank them without suggesting it may have been a waste of time' (p. 53).

Related to the issue of snowball technique and consent was the position of the person who linked me up with a potential participant. Here, power relations may have played a role. One of the women participants I requested to assist me with contacting others was a faculty dean. She suggested that I interview a particular woman who had been to an HIV and AIDS course in South Africa together with others. The dean (whom I call Prof. Nyaboke) believed that her suggested contact would provide me with deeper insights on HIV and AIDS from this course in addition to her own experiences. Prof. Nyaboke called the woman while I was still in her office but she was not available. She promised she would follow up on her and also gave me her cell phone number. I called this woman (whom I call Dr. Nkirote) many times but did not get through. Although I left a few messages on her phone, she did not return my calls.

After failing to reach Dr. Nkirote on the phone, I made a decision to stop looking for her. I also thought it helpful not to mention this to Prof. Nyaboke because I did not want her to influence Dr. Nkirote's decision. I was surprised when Dr. Nkirote called me almost two months later, informing me that she had received a call from her dean about my research and she was then ready for the interview. This was an ethical dilemma for me because I was not sure if she had done this out of her own free will or because a senior person had requested her. Yet I could not turn her offer down as I felt that would not only be rude, but I would also be letting down my friend who had tried to assist me to access this woman.

I was conscious of what Miller and Bell (2002) argue regarding consent that "whichever approach is adopted, the motives around why some people become participants and others resist should

concern the researcher and be documented in a research diary" (p. 56). This is what I did as I could sense some resistance, although not very clearly.

However, after Dr. Nkirote offered to meet me, my decision to go ahead with the interview was informed by the argument presented by Alderson and Morrow (2004) that consent may take time as participants evaluate the information on the research and then make a decision. I recall going to this interview not sure if we would have a good and useful conversation. To my surprise, she was extremely open and helpful and I can only assume that she had taken her time to think about the research or she may have simply been busy as she told me, when she apologised for being unable to meet me earlier. This made me feel better as I had read of other feminist researchers' experiences with gatekeepers and how they could influence whether women participants felt able to speak about their experiences, more so on sensitive issues (Miller, 1998). I did not view Prof. Nyaboke as a gatekeeper in the strict sense, but her position as a dean was an issue of concern.

In many of the other cases, I was careful to avoid asking contact people to provide the details of my study. I would ask to be given contact details of potential interviewees instead so that I could make contact with them directly. This meant that a lot of time was spent on the telephone explaining the nature of my study to potential participants. These conversations, though unique for each participant, would begin with some basic information about the study and myself:

My name is Nyokabi; I am a lecturer at the Catholic University, currently taking my doctoral studies at the University of London. I am calling to request you for an interview in a research project I am carrying out for my PhD. We shall talk about your experiences with HIV and AIDS at a personal level and also your views on how your university is responding to the epidemic. This will be a very informal and relaxed interview at a place most convenient for you preferably where we will not be disturbed... (My research notes, September 10, 2004).

It was during this introduction that I asked them whether I could record the interview.

Mentioning that I was a lecturer was an important part of my introduction especially when approaching senior academics and administrators as they viewed me as a colleague. I realised that in a sensitive topic, being viewed as 'one of the participants' was helpful (Bergen, 1993). I could tell the interest that part of my introduction elicited from my potential participants. Being a doctoral student also seems to have been interesting especially to those colleagues who were either pursuing their own doctorates or were planning to embark on the same. Getting a doctorate is seen as an important and rare opportunity in Kenya, especially for women, hence this aspect also accorded me some respect. Tang (2002) discusses similar experiences with interviewing academic women in China, where being a doctoral student was treated with some respect.

Subsequent to the telephone conversations, some people would make an appointment with me immediately, while others asked me to call them at a later date. Some declined with the excuse that they were busy or just politely said they would get back to me. I did not expect anyone to call me back and none did, so I took that as unwillingness to participate, and I did not call them again. In the next section, I discuss the interviews showing how power relations became apparent in the process of interviewing, especially with senior people.

The Interview Context

Throughout all the interviews, I tried the best I could to allow the participants to talk about only what they felt free and comfortable with. The unstructured and conversational nature of my interviews allowed this to happen easily. I was conscious of the fact that approaching participants directly required a great deal of skill on my side to develop rapport with strangers. I was however careful not to use this skill to exploit the participants into talking about issues they would otherwise regret (Duncombe and Jessop, 2002 discuss the issue of rapport in details). Developing rapport became a necessary skill in approaching strangers directly and in negotiating consent.

Where the interviews were carried out was an important factor (Tang, 2002) given that our discussions dwelt on private issues. During the pilot study, I learnt that carrying out interviews in offices posed the problem of facing many disruptions like telephone calls and people coming in and out. In one of the pilot interviews held in an office, the telephone and a few visitors disturbed us. Two of the pilot interviews were held in a quiet restaurant and I thought this would be a good option if the participants would be agreeable to it.

About the interview context, Wragg (2002) observes that when people are interviewed in familiar places, they may be too comfortable, which may lead to giving some 'false' information. Neutral ground can be best for both the interviewer and the interviewee especially if they are of similar social status or where the interviewee is of higher social status as in many of my interviews.

Negotiating the place to carry out the interviews turned out to be a power-related issue. The more senior the interviewee, the more difficult it was for me to select the venue of the interview, a factor I had not envisaged initially. During the pilot study, I was able to negotiate for a neutral place with two fairly senior people. I had met one of the pilot interviewees in a gender conference mentioned earlier on, while the other one was a colleague and a friend. Hence, the power relations were slightly different as they viewed me as an equal, despite our formal professional positions.

During the main study, it became apparent that the more senior the interviewees, the more difficult it would be to negotiate the choice of an interview venue. I realised that, as Bergen (1993) notes, when her interviewees 'hosted' the interviews, they were more in control of the situation and they exercised much more power. Bergen found this to be good for the women in her interviews as they were in the more familiar position of hostess and this made them much more relaxed. This was helpful for her study where being a researcher accorded her a higher social status. My situation was different since being a student and a junior to many of my respondents in age, qualifications, position at the university, and in some cases economic status, led me to have less power to control the situation. It was more difficult for me when the participants 'hosted' the interviews because they were in control while I felt powerless.

A total of eight interviews were carried out in a place we both negotiated and agreed, mainly in private clubs that were good for privacy. The rest were held in the interviewees' offices and two were done in their houses. Some of the interviewees chose to be interviewed away from their offices because they did not have their own private offices, which was an indication of their positions in the university. Many of these were close to me in either age or position in the university.

On the issue of age, Reynolds (2002) observes that she too was intimidated by the wide generation gap between her and some of the women in her study. This generation difference can render one powerless, especially coming from a social context like mine where I have been brought up to be respectful of elders.

Some of the questions and dilemmas that I faced when I carried out interviews in people's offices and houses were: Could I suggest we sit in a quiet place or ask them to turn off their mobile phones? Could I ask them to lock the office doors? Some people locked the doors on noticing that the disturbance was too much. But a few others allowed the disturbances and there was nothing I could do about it as they were in their own offices or homes (see above on Dr. Muasia's interview). For those with whom I had lunch or tea after the interview, we ended up with some enriching off-the record conversations whose benefits I discuss elsewhere in this chapter.

I invited all my research participants (except the VC) to lunch or tea as a way of saying 'thank you' and many accepted the offer. I found the lunch or teatime to be a helpful way of unwinding especially after some discussions on emotional matters.

In the offices of more senior men and women who had secretaries, there were fewer disturbances as the secretaries handled visitors and telephones calls. However, there was the question of mobile phones. When I interviewed women of my age and level or those with whom I had struck a good rapport, we were able to come to some agreements like putting off our mobile phones.

Age and rank in the university played a role in the amount of power that the respondents exercised in the control of the context (Lee, 2001; Tang, 2002; Thapar-Bjorkert and Henry, 2004). Thapar-Bjorkert and Henry (2004) challenge some feminist writing which has tended to focus on the power that the researcher has over the researched; for example, Acker, et al. (1991) caution researchers to take care not to make the research relationship an exploitative one assuming the power lies with the researcher. Acker et al. (1991) ignore the fact that in some situations, the researched can have some power over the researcher. In my study, being a researcher gave me a certain sense of power. However, the respondents too could control some factors like when and where to meet me, for how long, and what they could talk about.

The power of the interviewee in some cases had an impact on the interviews as we were sometimes interrupted and the flow of the discussions would be affected. This was apparent during the interview with the Vice Chancellor. The VC's office is viewed with high regard, especially in public universities. Before I could interview him, I had to wait for about three hours in an office far away from his. The person who escorted me to his office was a security officer. The security detail, the office size, décor and the size of the man were all quite intimidating. To further add to my powerlessness, after I explained my mission, he said he had only three minutes! Even before I could ask the first question, his cell phone rang and he asked me to excuse him. Again, the security officer escorted me out of the office. On my return, I could hardly follow my interview schedule, but just asked what I thought was important.

Tang (2002) writes about similar experiences when she interviewed senior academics in the UK and in China. Here, it was not just the sensitivity of the topic, but also the office, which is also sensitive. On that day, for example, there were very many union leaders of the support staff waiting outside to discuss an impending strike. The security was therefore on high alert. I needed to be patient and ready to change my interview accordingly, as I was at the mercy of a powerful and senior man. I felt humbled, and was not in control of the interview in the way I would have been. However, I was still able to gather some useful information. I sensed that, being an academic myself, although a junior one, I could have made the Vice Chancellor to give me the little time he did. I do not know if he would have given his precious time had I been 'just' a research student, and a woman.

It is important to note that although there were all these power issues, I found my interviews successful and they fulfilled my objectives. I managed to do this by making known to the interviewees what my research was about. Many of them showed interest in the study, as the quotation below indicates:

> Well, I think what you are doing is good because AIDS is here and when I go to class I usually tell my students that we all need to do something about this problem as it affects each one of us. So each one of us is in it and even if we are not infected we don't know what tomorrow holds. I hope you'll come up with something that will help us address this issue to help the students and us (Prof. Nyaboke, Weruini University).

I was also reflexive throughout the process and recognising some areas where we had common experiences, hence breaking any power barriers that may have existed (see also Chapter Eight).

In addition, the conversational and relaxed nature of the interviews helped many of the interviewees to relax and reveal information and express their feelings without much reservation.

In addition to the challenges that surrounded the issues of access, consent and where the interviews were held, which I have discussed so far, there were some ethical issues in the interview itself, which I discuss next.

Interviews as Therapy

I embarked on this research while aware (from the pilot study, from my reading, and from talking to other feminist researchers) that some people would talk about personal issues and there was a possibility of some of them looking at the sessions as therapeutic. However, I appreciated that a research interview need not become a therapy session (Mason, 2002).

Nevertheless, talking about sensitive issues has been viewed by some feminist researchers as prompting an understanding of past events for themselves, in ways that the interviewees may not have done before and which may play a therapeutic role (Birch and Miller, 2000; Opie, 1992; Skeggs, 1994). Birch and Miller (2000), for example, write about their experiences of researching sensitive topics where the women in their studies confessed that in talking about private and sensitive matters, they were able to reflect and come to a better understanding of past experiences in different and sometimes more positive ways that promoted a changed sense of self. Some of the participants in these studies told the researchers that they had found the interviews therapeutic. Many of the women in my study said that some of the information they had given me had not even been talked about openly in their own families. The free talk, after the tape recorder had been switched off, also seemed to play a therapeutic role for them and also for myself, as I explain in section further in this chapter.

Birch and Miller (2000), however, note that there is a danger of the participants placing the researcher in the role of therapist or counsellor, which they may not be qualified for or would be unable to fulfil. They recommend that researchers should be prepared to support participants in accessing professional help if required rather than finding themselves in a situation they (the researchers) cannot handle. My interviewees did not directly ask for information about where they could seek help. There were instances when we had long discussions after the interview and it was during such conversations that we talked about where further help could be sought. Several others called me long after the interviews enquiring about issues ranging from some academic aspects of the research to where they could seek help on matters related to HIV and AIDS. I have helped wherever I could by referring them to relevant offices. However, I too had to deal with the effects the interviews had on me, which I discuss next.

The Researcher's Support of Self

In social research involving sensitive issues, the emotional strain has potential risks for both the researcher and the participants. But, generally, much attention is given to the impact on the participants (Corden et al., 2005). Having keenly followed the experiences of other researchers who have studied sensitive topics (Chatzifotiou, 2000; Dunn, 1991; Hubbard et al., 2001; Mauthner, 2000; Rotham, 1986), I did not want to be caught unawares having to deal with emotional strain and stress. Chatzifotiou (2000), for example, discusses how she interviewed battered women without realising that she too would deal with a whole set of emotions as the women in her study told her their painful stories.

On the same issue, Corden et al. (2005) discuss the need for researchers to be professionally prepared before embarking on researching emotional topics. They note the value of working closely where a team of researchers is involved, with debriefing meetings and discussions. I had no access to professional help or support of a team; hence, I had to be creative to keep myself 'safe'. My research journal and my earlier training in social work became useful in helping me cope with the painful experiences expressed in the interviews.

In total, I listened to over 20 hours of stories from women, some of which were full of pain, anger, regret, blame and guilt. I realised that the only way I could manage to work with this was to carry out only one interview a day and a maximum of four interviews each week. There were weeks when I would have only one or even no interview at all. Only twice in the whole time did I have two interviews in one day. This was necessitated by change of appointments by the interviewees. These breaks were healthy for me as I gave myself time to reflect on the conversations; on the impact they were having on me and indeed prepare myself psychologically for the next one.

I did not need to consult a counsellor as I had earlier thought I might. However, I took good care of myself through regular exercises (yoga was especially helpful), taking walks in the evenings, treating myself to a full body massage every month and peer debriefing with the two close professional colleagues that I have mentioned in Chapter Three.

In addition to taking care of myself, I also found that the discussions with the women played a therapeutic role for me. On several occasions when the 'official' interview was over, the women and I had relaxed conversations. Many of them talked about other experiences in their lives and in some cases we would talk for over two hours after the interviews. I found these conversations after the main interviews empowering and a source of encouragement. On this I am encouraged by the thoughts of Acker, et al. (1991) about feminist research:

> ...at the same time women researchers were developing analyses of their own locations in the larger socio economic structure, for in some fundamental ways their positions were and are similar to those of

their subjects. As women, they too may have husbands and children they too keep house as well as work, they too have to cope with sexism in their daily lives. Thus sociology for women has emancipator possibilities for the researchers as well as the researched, for as women researchers we have also been unheard within the main sociological traditions (p. 135).

The reflexive methodology allowed this sharing to occur easily. I have continued communicating with some of these women by email. This closeness has, however, brought some ethical challenges when it comes to the issue of researching a sensitive topic with people in my network, colleagues, whom I will continue to meet in forums, in some of which I will be talking about this research. I discuss these two issues in the following sections.

Researching Colleagues

Researching colleagues, especially on the issue of HIV and AIDS, has created a certain sense of discomfort in me. Shahidian (2001) points out the dilemma that he too faced in relation to researching his own ethnic group and peers. Some researchers like Brannen (1988) suggest that it is better for participants if they do not meet the researcher again where private issues have been disclosed. In Brannen's (1988) study, respondents were consoled by the one-off nature of their encounter because there was less fear of meeting again. This was not the case with my participants who were my colleagues and I continued to meet them after the research. Even as the research was still in progress, I met some of the participants in two conferences where I was talking about my research findings, an issue I return to later in this chapter.

There is a dilemma about the appropriate ways of ending research relationship and then have a 'normal relationship' with people who belong to the same network. Skeggs (1995) acknowledges the challenges that face a researcher because of the many different kinds of relationships established in the course of the research. This is especially challenging for a feminist researcher whose ontology and epistemology demand "a need to reciprocate, not exploit, not abuse power, to care, empower and to be honest" (Skeggs, 1995: 194).

I had reflected on this issue of ending research relationships and had several conversations with my supervisor about it. My supervisor and I agreed that it would be helpful to end all the relationships professionally and carefully. I did this by sending all the respondents 'thank you' cards after each interview. For those that I met later on, I avoided referring to the interviews unless they asked how I was getting along. Similarly, Morley (1999), acknowledges that this is a good way of dealing with interviewees after a research undertaking is over.

I interviewed one woman who goes to the same health club that went to. Initially, there seemed to be some discomfort because she is one of those who disclosed matters that she said were not talked about even in her family. After she received my 'thank you' note, she seemed more relaxed because we had put that particular 'research relationship' to a close. We moved on to discuss other issues not related to the research whenever we met.

As noted earlier in this chapter, some women continued to consult me on my methodology as they said they liked the conversational nature of the interviews and that they would like to adapt it in their work. I was happy to assist whenever I could. However, even after these relationships were safely and sensitively terminated, another dilemma that I continue to grapple with is the ethical dissemination of the research findings, which I discuss next.

Dissemination of Findings

In a study of sensitive issues, there are always some ethical dilemmas that face the researcher when it comes to writing up and indeed disseminating the findings. Shahidian (2001) argues that when it comes to writing about a group of people, one may not remain completely objective in recounting their life-experiences. Besides remaining faithful to the stories, some of which are truly deep and personal, I am also struggling with the question of guaranteeing anonymity about the issues we discussed. I promised all my participants that nowhere will their real names and those of their institutions be used in the final report. However, this has proved to be difficult as the following incident shows.

In the conference I mentioned at the start of this chapter (CHE and UNESCO, 2004), I was given a session in which to present the impressions I had from the research. Among other issues, I spoke about an interview with a faculty dean at the Holy Ghost University. The dean's response to the impact of HIV and AIDS in his university was as indicated in the following quotation:

> No, we haven't had any people infected with HIV and AIDS, either the faculty or students. One, because we are a Christian university who go by certain values that everybody is signed up to and before anyone comes in, they must be tested and they must show commitment to Christian values and so when they are here they know that certain behaviour will not be acceptable. So that is where we are... (Dr Kivuu, HG).

This seems to have touched a raw nerve in the person chairing this session who, to my surprise, was a professor from Holy Ghost University, actually the Deputy Vice Chancellor (DVC). I had written a letter requesting to interview the DVC, but he had instead referred me to Dr. Kivuu (quoted above). Presently, when he spoke after my presentation, he asked me through the microphone: "Are you the Nyokabi who had written to me requesting for an interview?" I was in a fix. How could I answer him when I had promised anonymity (of individuals and their institutions) to all the people I had interviewed some of whom were among the audience? I shook my head to mean I was not the person he was referring to. This was an ethical dilemma when trying to talk in a conference about research findings, which are viewed as sensitive.

Later on in August, 2005, I received an email from one of my interviewees who was part of a team editing articles for a journal. He was asking me to send him a chapter based on my research. Again, I found myself faced with the dilemma of sending him my work where he was one of the interviewees. I was concerned about his reaction to the interpretations I made, especially because he represented management. Nonetheless, I knew that this was a great opportunity for me to have my work published in an international publication. I realised that I would continuously be faced by such feelings, yet it was no use carrying out a study if the findings are not publicly disseminated. I sent the paper, and I learnt from the same man that it was accepted for the publication.

Summary and Conclusion

In this chapter, I have shown that there are a number of key areas where difficult decisions are required in designing social research on HIV and AIDS, not least with regard to the ethics of intrusion into sensitive areas and the devising of means for securing reliable information. Other researchers in this area of HIV and AIDS (for example, Bujra and Baylies 2000) have argued that research on a topic relating to the private domain of social relations raises issues regarding access to data and questions about its quality. Hence, I have argued throughout this chapter that the study of sensitive topics presents certain challenges to the researcher that are best thought about before the study itself commences and continue to be reflected on throughout the research process.

I found that the pilot study played a crucial role in preparing me for some of the surprises that emerged in the main fieldwork. I have also learnt that a researcher needs to be flexible at all times and be ready to change accordingly as much of what is laid out in the research design does not always fit with the actual situation in the field. I am glad that I had prepared some ethical guidelines before starting the data collection, which became a useful reference throughout the fieldwork (see Appendix 2).

= 5

The Feminist Perspectives and Concepts Used in this Study

Introduction

The present study utilises a feminist perspective, which stresses that the relationship between men and women is that of inequality. The perspective connects the various elements of women's position in society (Leonard, 2001). It acknowledges that the power, which operates in personal relationships of parenthood and marriage, and informally with colleagues at work, is also political and it allows issues which matter to women to be raised, understood and collectively challenged (Leonard, 2001). I find this definition of feminist perspective by Leonard appropriate for the purposes of this study. However, I still need to explain what I understand by the term 'feminism'.

Feminism is itself a diverse concept, which according to Ramazanoglu and Holland (2002):

> Covers a diversity of beliefs, practices and politics, and these overlap and interact with other beliefs, practices and politics. For every generalization that one can make about feminism it is possible to find 'feminists' who do not fit, or who do not want to fit (p.5).

Given this diversity, I decided that in the Kenyan context, where my study was located, feminism generally indicates the advocacy for women's rights. These rights, on which Kenyan feminists are still working, are in the areas of education, political representation, health, sexuality, motherhood, legal rights, property ownership and working conditions (see Chapter Two).

From a rights' perspective, feminism provided me with the concepts used to analyse the experiences narrated in this research. My use of a feminist perspective is justified by the existence in Kenyan universities of gender relations that are unjust and oppressive (Onsongo, 2005). This research is one tool that can be used to change these relations and practices in the university sector and provide other researchers with language and data to explore this area further. In Chapter Six, I explore how the university sector in Kenya and in much of the world is seen to be oppressive of women.

The five concepts (patriarchy, discourse, the personal as political, care and silence) discussed in this chapter emerged from the literature review and also from the data. The process has been iterative as issues emerged from reading and then appeared in the field and were checked again in the literature as I have discussed later in this chapter. Although 'personal is political' is a feminist slogan rather than a concept, it was a recurring theme both in the literature and the interviews, especially about care work done by women. Hence, it is a basic concept and is included in this chapter, and it is used to analyse women's responsibilities as a result of HIV and AIDS and the impact of these on their public professional lives (Chapter Seven).

In this chapter, I explain my feminist journey, outlining how I came to choose to work with a feminist perspective, while also appreciating that the women I interviewed may not have taken a similar journey. However, I see this study in itself as a way of sensitising them about issues they may have either chosen to be silent about or were not 'allowed' to talk about.

It is the aim of this chapter to provide a discussion about some aspects of feminist theory that have helped me to appreciate the complex ways in which women's gender identities can become silenced and invisible in institutional discourse. It needs to be stressed that this chapter contains an inevitably theoretical discussion, which is simply setting out the main elements of the framework that provides the basis of the chapters to follow. It needs to be read in conjunction with subsequent chapters, which in their presentation and analysis of the data further clarify the concepts discussed here.

My Feminist Journey

I carried out the present feminist research at a point in my life when I felt comfortable to be termed a feminist. By using my life experience as a justification for my use of a feminist perspective, I have borrowed from Weiner (1994) who notes:

> The work we do and the perspectives that we hold are the products of the interrelationship between the personal biography, our place in the social structure, and the cultural milieu and historical period in which we live (p.10).

My feminist journey, which I briefly outline here, needs to be read as a conscious selection of certain events and influences in my life that help explain the origins and developments of the ideas I present in this thesis.

My first encounter with issues of discrimination and injustice that women face started when I was a young girl. I grew up in Kamirithu village, Kiambu County, where women performed almost all the domestic chores regardless of whether their husbands were gainfully employed or not. My mother was a 'housewife', while my father was a teacher. (I put housewife in inverted commas because most of her work was away from the house.) My mother's working day started at 5 a.m. and ended after midnight when the rest of the family had gone to bed. She bore 10 children, 9 of whom survived (one passed on at an early age of 3 months). The child she lost, who was her second child, also happened to have been a boy. This loss of a boy child was seen to be a tremendous misfortune by the whole community. My mother therefore had to bear 5 other girls before she could eventually give birth to her only son. Two other girls were born after the boy; maybe my parents hoped they would bear a second son. I therefore learnt quite early that boys were seen as very important, but I was never sure why this was so until later when I joined Women's Studies.

Although I witnessed imbalances in gender roles at this early age, I did not feel directly discriminated against or treated differently because I was a girl all through my school years, until I joined university. It was when I was a university student that a lecturer approached me for a sexual favour promising that he would give me good marks. I somehow managed to say no and we maintained a friendship that has lasted to this date. He is now a senior academic at a leading Kenyan university. I am still concerned about issues of sexual harassment in universities, an issue to which I return later in this section. The argument that female students deliberately seduce lecturers hoping to get favours cannot hold any water given that the lecturer is always at a position of power which must be used responsibly.

Before I joined academic work, I worked with NGOs and I did not experience any form of discrimination as a woman. The first discrimination that I became aware of as an employee was when I started working at a university. This university had a medical policy, under which the dependants of male staff members were covered, while those of female staff members were not. Female staff members complained that this was discrimination, but the university administration maintained that it was not their responsibility to look after our families as long as we had husbands.

I discussed this discrimination issue with other female colleagues, but none of them were willing to take the issue further. They were all unhappy with the situation, but they feared that they could lose their jobs if they complained. The absence of a channel through which we could air our views was a discouraging factor. We were also very few women at that time and people were more concerned about job security. We were then on one-year contracts and few could afford not to have their contracts renewed every year.

I felt very uncomfortable with this situation and decided to talk to the Deputy Vice Chancellor (DVC) Finance who was in charge of staff benefits. He still maintained that it was not the university's responsibility to look after our families as long as we had husbands. I negotiated that my family be included in the policy and agreed to meet the costs through deductions from my salary. This was accepted although in the end, the deductions were not made. In the meantime I felt demoralised and I lost interest in most of the university activities. I considered one of the options mentioned by Adler et al. (1993) of leaving the profession and pursuing other careers that would give me more job satisfaction. However, I chose to remain in the university since the flexibility of the working hours for a junior lecturer was convenient, especially because I had a young family and also needed to further my studies.

In 1999, the dean asked me whether I would be interested in attending a workshop on Women and Management in Higher Education, in Lagos, Nigeria. I was delighted because it was going to be a break from the monotony of my work. I accepted, but he said he could not confirm until I had consulted my husband whether this would be okay (for me to be away from home for one week!) I told him that my husband would be okay with it, without having contacted him. A woman colleague and I attended the workshop, which was sponsored by the Association of Commonwealth Universities (ACU).

During this workshop, I was able to analyse my feelings better and to understand fully that what I was going through was not unique to me. Other women had gone through similar experiences. This conference contributed significantly towards my interest in feminism and women's studies.

In our plan of action at the end of the conference, we agreed that we would begin by sensitising all lecturers and administrators on gender issues in our institution. We held a one-day workshop that was attended by 45 participants, both lectures and administrators, including the academic dean and the finance director. At the end of the day it was clear that we had achieved our objective because the participants drew up a plan of action about how to make the university more women-friendly. Later on, I was able to meet the finance officer and he agreed in principle to revise the medical policy to have women covered with their families. This was indeed implemented for all the women.

Another discriminatory experience arose when I was signing my study leave contract to take up a Masters degree in Women and Management in Higher Education (WMHE) at the Institute of Education, University of London, funded by the ACU. Having become aware of the subtle discriminatory practices that women may face in the academy, I was alert to practices that I may not have noticed earlier on. I realised that the allowances paid to staff on study leave were not the same for all, but were to be negotiated depending on family circumstances. I learnt that as a married woman, I would get less than a male colleague who was also leaving for studies. At that point I did nothing to challenge the situation because I did not want to jeopardise my study leave.

My MA programme in the UK became the real catalyst to my becoming a full feminist. Even though I had become aware of the discrimination that women face in my university and in my culture, I was still very cautious about calling myself a feminist. I had come to believe that feminism was a foreign term that could only be used by and about women who did not like men, those who were divorced or who were angry about life in general. This perception about feminists and feminism had been created by the Kenyan political leadership during the years of Moi's rule, as I note in Chapter Two, and was also written about by Maathai (2006).

During my MA course, I became more familiar with feminists and began to understand their views. It was then that I started to embrace feminism fully and to develop the courage to call myself a feminist.

Due to my position as a feminist, which was no longer a secret in my university, I became unpopular with my male colleagues because of my stand on issues affecting women on campus. Some students had talked to the then Dean of Students (also a woman) and myself about a male lecturer who was demanding sex in exchange for good grades. When we raised this in a meeting, we were accused of wanting to malign the names of our male colleagues and of inciting students.

In 2002, with a group of three other women (three of us had been though the WMHE MA and the fourth one had been to the Lagos workshop mentioned earlier), we organised a regional WMHE workshop in my university. There were also five participants from our university. For the first time, I saw a change of attitude towards gender issues by these women. They started mentioning a need for us to form a support group where we could discuss issues that were affecting us.

Unfortunately, this did not materialise because all three of us who had planned the workshop left the country soon afterwards for our doctorates. However, it was from this workshop that my interests on the topic of this thesis began (see Chapter One).

The above workshop accorded us a great deal of publicity, which was problematic because in my case, my head of department seemed threatened. Afterwards, my efforts to get a doctoral scholarship were frustrated by my head of department. He conspired with the dean to deny me the opportunity to be funded by the university or even to be recommended for funding.

I later experienced sexual harassment from a visiting professor. He tried to force a kiss from me in his office and he asked me if I would have an affair with him. I reported the matter to the VC who called the professor and I to his office. I was asked me to forgive the professor in the Christian spirit. The professor however denied any wrongdoing. He said that he had only hugged me the 'West African way', which was common amongst colleagues and commented that he was surprised that I had been offended.

Miroiu (2003) refers to such behaviour as 'friendly harassment'. This kind of harassment is defined as "behaviour that is apparently innocent and benign, but actually creates discomfort, intimidation and inhibition" (p. 24). These incidents continued to make me unpopular and consequently I was not recommended for a scholarship through my university. I was helped by the 'Gender Equity in Higher Education' project based at the Institute of Education, which offered me a scholarship to take up my PhD. However, the university informed me they would not give me study leave although they had initially indicated leave would be granted.

The journey I have described here chronicles both the discrimination I have been subjected to, and my growing awareness and understanding of the effects of patriarchy. So I use a feminist perspective in my study, aware that the women I interviewed may not have gone through the development of a similar understanding. I hoped that the interviews would make some of the women to begin to question the patriarchal and power structures in their institutions and decide to plan for change. I address these issues further in the data chapters and in my final reflections of the research process in Chapter Ten. In the next section, I discuss further why I felt comfortable to work with a feminist perspective as an African woman.

Why I Chose a Feminist Perspective

As an African woman, I identify with feminism while aware of some controversy that this concept has elicited among African women (Kolawole, 1997). Some African women writers have found the term 'feminism' foreign, while some have embraced it altogether. Kolawole (1997), for example, notes that:

> A major problem emerges from throwing one's voice unless the African woman is firmly determined not to allow her voice to be submerged by existing feminist discourse. While some are assertive in identifying with feminism, others are cautious, while others will have nothing to do with feminism as it is presented from the West (p. 7).

Kolawole (1997) further notes that African women who accept feminism, whether black or Western, risk being viewed as parrots:

> As opposed to being creative and creating our own discourses...some women see concepts such as African feminism and Black feminism as identical to singing African songs from the belly of the beast (p.10).

In Kenya, there have also been sentiments that anything to do with feminism is foreign (Kuria, 2003). I have been told on several occasions that I only call myself a feminist because I have been brainwashed in the West.

There are indeed some African feminists who have faced threats and condemnation because of their position. One such example is provided by McFadden (2003) who describes how she was deported from Zimbabwe in the mid 1990s:

> The government issued me with a deportation order, in which accusations of my betrayal of the 'Zimbabwean culture' and 'family values' featured prominently. I was identified as a lesbian (and therefore automatically vilified), on the grounds that I wrote about women's rights...and because I defended rights of gays and lesbians... the fact that I am a relatively contended heterosexual was forgotten or ignored...my feminist stance was defined as "dangerous" (p. 53).

McFadden (2003) further observes that even those in the women's movement in Zimbabwe remained silent when the government was harassing her. This silence could have been due to their own fears of supporting a position seen by their government to be against their culture, even though they may have wanted to support her. I discuss silence further in this chapter, and it is a theme that runs through the entire study.

Other African feminists have cited experiences of being condemned and misunderstood (e.g., Tamale, 2005) but this has not stopped them from carrying out feminist work even if they may not label themselves as such. One Kenyan woman who has fully embraced the term 'feminism' is Dr. Wanjiku Kabira (see Kuria, 2003). Dr Kabira argues that African women need to embrace feminism as it provides them with a platform to fight injustices against women, which many African men condone or simply ignore (Kuria, 2003). Similarly, Kolawole (1997) quotes Abena Busia, a Ghanaian writer, as having noted in an interview:

> I am comfortable with the term 'feminism'. If we concede the term feminism, we've lost a power struggle. As a strategy, we might be conceding grounds that we shouldn't...feminism is an ideological

praxis that gives us a series of multiple strategies (of reading, of analysis) and what those strategies have in common is that woman matters (Kolawole, 1997: 8).

I adopted Abena Busia's position because feminism provided me with strategies for reading and analysing women's experiences with the AIDS pandemic in Kenyan universities. To arrive at this decision of using a feminist perspective to theorise Kenyan university women's experiences with HIV and AIDS, I had been through various experiences that exposed me to women's issues. These included the WMHE workshop in Lagos, the Masters degree, and later on, the workshop held in Nairobi.

It was after the Nairobi workshop that I started thinking about research that is book is about. On joining doctoral studies, I spent the first year reading on HIV and AIDS, gender, women issues, feminist theory and higher education. This literature helped me to finalise my research question, ready for testing in a pilot study. From the pilot study, I rephrased my research question as new issues emerged and others were confirmed. From further reading after the pilot study, I refined my question and went for the main data collection, which lasted for seven months.

During this period, I attended some conferences and continued engaging with literature and discussions with colleagues on issues that were emerging. It was from this iterative process that the theoretical framework that I adapted for this study was developed, which made me to work on three premises:

(1) That a category of women, clearly differentiated from men exists;

(2) That women have some common conditions of gendered existence, despite the social and cultural divisions between them; and,

(3) That women suffer universal injustices (Ramazanoglu & Holland, 2002).

My arguments in the following chapters of this book clarify these three points in relation to senior university women.

Challenges of Choosing Which Feminist Positions to Work With

From the onset of this research project, the question about which aspects of feminist perspectives that I needed to embrace was central. I have found the breadth of feminist theorising quite intimidating, especially because I had been in this discourse for only five years. In addition, almost all the literature available in this area is 'foreign' to me as the majority of the writers are Western.

On this issue of 'foreign' literature, Dube (2004) argues that Western education can sometimes leave "African scholars feeling lame and impotent because much of what they learn is totally foreign to the African context" (p. 110). However, the feminist theoretical issues with which I identify are relevant to my African-Kenyan background.

In addition to my dilemma about which perspectives to adapt, it was clear to me from the onset, that my study would be set within the context of a feminist theoretical framework which illuminates the significance of gender in society (Chatzifotiou, 2000: 276). Feminist research needs to be informed by feminist theory because "other theoretical traditions downplay the interaction of gender and power" (Reinharz, 1992: 249).

Having considered the various feminist stances available, which are not only daunting but also sometimes confusing, I associated myself with Leonard's (2001) observation about the challenges that newcomers into feminist research are faced with:

> ...a daunting literature...it is all too often verbose and jargonised... problematising seemingly simple words and pairings, and drawing on disciplines with which you may not be at all familiar... sometimes the fact of 'subordination' is missing and women's agency is seen to override any contexts or constraints (p. 193).

Leonard's observation echoes my feelings about much of Western feminist theorising, which has sometimes failed to identify with the pressing problems facing Kenyan women. For me, gender equality only makes sense when it looks at women and men as distinct categories so that even when thinking of gender sensitive policies, it is ensured that these are policies, which would recognise that society is made up of men and women who require a different focus.

Scott (1988; 1990) observes that, "power is constructed and must be challenged from the ground of difference" and that "difference does not preclude equality" (Scott, 1998: 48; Scott, 1990: 138). She further notes that, "equality is not the elimination of difference, and difference does not preclude equality (Scott, 1990:137-38). If women are placed in a 'general "human" identity', then the particularity of women's experiences may get lost (Scott, 1988: 45). We would be back to the days when everything was seen from the man's point of view.

Recognising differences between men and women helps to keep women visible. However, appreciating gender differences without moving into absolutes and essentialism (e.g., that every woman wants to get married or to be a mother or wants to care for the sick) can help women to see the need to focus on their differences while still negotiating for equality. I support the position that equality between men and women can be achieved if their differences are appreciated and included in policy and practice.

I noted that there are different feminist perspectives and strands available; for example, African, Christian, black, liberal, socialist, radical and cultural. I therefore decided to work with those perspectives that best fitted my study. This decision was informed by Maynard (1995) when she argues that feminists need to take a 'middle-range' approach in their theorising rather than associating with certain grand theories.

Similarly, Hughes (2002) notes that:

> While there are relatively standard distinctions in the feminist literature, there are considerable overlaps between the positions that individual theorists may take up within each of these distinctions... (p. 82).

I use those aspects of feminist perspectives that allow me to look into "neglected aspects of women's lives, grounded in their own experiences and from a particular theoretical and methodological perspective that we call feminist despite the breadth of the term" (Birch et al., 2002: 3). I have drawn upon a range of approaches and ideas rather than identifying with one category or strand of feminism which Maynard (1995) notes:

> Encourages the idea that a particular writer's understanding of women's subordination and inferior position can simply be inferred from the characteristics generally ascribed to that category (p. 264).

From the different feminist approaches, I gained a clear understanding of concepts that are central to my research. These are: patriarchy, discourse, 'the personal is political', care and silence.

Patriarchy

The central question that this study sought to answer was whether two Kenyan universities have taken into consideration the experiences of senior women staff in their responses to HIV and AIDS. This question is based on the assumption that, for institutional policies and programmes to change, the systems and structures that govern them need to be well understood, and revised, if necessary.

The discussion in Chapter Two has shown that workplaces in Kenya are still governed by some deeply rooted patriarchal power structures. I use the concept of 'patriarchy' as defined by McCloskey (1999) to mean:

> A system of social structures and practices in which men dominate, oppress and exploit women…the manifestation and institutionalisation of male dominance over women and children in the family and the extension of male dominance over women in society in general. It means that men hold power in all important institutions in society (cited in Oakley 2002: 216).

In Kenya, as I discussed in Chapter Two and as it emerged from the data, it is men who hold most positions of power in the institutions of family, religion, politics and the workplace. Even when women hold positions of power, it is a struggle to overcome the societal attitudes that they too can perform as well as men (Maathai, 2006). Due to patriarchy, the Kenyan society organises its affairs to cater for and sustain male supremacy over women (Nzomo, 2003b).

Patriarchy in Kenya has its roots in long established traditions of male dominance, which have made the male perspective, to be the social perspective (Maathai, 2006). HIV and AIDS have exposed dangers of many of these societies' practices over time. Patriarchy is one of them, as Siplon (2005) notes:

> Patriarchy, with all its attendant denial of resources, respect, and decision- making ability for women, represents one such form of managing power and relationships that has become deadly in the era of AIDS (p.17).

Universities are part of wider patriarchal structures, which make them subject to external economic, social, cultural and political pressures, even when they have control over their internal organisation. This internal organisation of universities tends to be seen by players as natural; hence, it cannot be questioned.

The hierarchy of structures, which characterises many, if not all universities, appears firm and unchangeable (Mabokela, 2003; Probert, 2005). Just like other institutions like the family, the state and religion, the people in these institutions have learnt to accept their positions and roles as given, hardly questioning the set rules and regulations. It can be argued that the relations between men and women in the workplace have been set by the social structure, which has put women in a subordinate position to that of men.

Delphy and Leonard (1992) argue that men get to benefit from the patriarchal social structure that keeps women in subordinate positions. Women serve men right from the domestic front to the workplace. Thus, women who may question or challenge patriarchy are viewed as deviants. Delphy and Leonard (1992) note that:

> Men also owe their occupational position, however well they treat their women colleagues, to the discrimination, which women suffer in employment. An individual man cannot renounce his position. He can merely choose not to take active advantage of existing privileges to get more. But very few men do in practice forgo accepting promotion to allow a woman to get it, or agree to full domestic role sharing, or full sex parity – though a few have been prepared to accept more modest moves towards equality (p. 261-2).

As the above statement suggests, although men may not as individuals actively help to keep women down and keep away their agendas, many of them do not question the status quo. I see universities as operating in this kind of patriarchal structure, where the majority of those at the top of the hierarchy are men. Even if the men are not against gender equality, they do nothing to change the situation. Some women, on the other hand, have learnt to take their life situations as God-given and hence they do not see the need to question the structures (see Chapter Seven).

By using the concept of patriarchy as a way of understanding how the two universities were operating, I am drawn to Kanter's (1977) argument that to improve the situation of women in organisations, it is important to understand the basic organisational and structural issues. These include the constraints imposed by roles and the effects of opportunity, power and numbers operating in these organisations.

Kanter (1997) notes that, "attention to these issues would require organisations – not people – to change" (p. 261). There may be no harm in having programmes that change women, making them more assertive as managers, and more effective communicators, among others. However, these need to go hand in hand with a critique of the patriarchal systems and structures (Kanter, 1977).

My wish in carrying out this study was to challenge the Kenyan university system to move away from patriarchal structures and provide equal opportunities for all employees. This study sought to provide a framework where the stakeholders in Kenyan universities would begin to see the need to put in place systems that embrace individuals as whole human beings so that their workplace caters for both their private and personal lives.

The language, debates and schools of thought used in universities also contribute to shape the structures, systems, policies and programmes of these institutions. In order for me to interpret and analyse women's experiences, I needed to understand the debates that were dominant in the two universities as far as HIV and AIDS was concerned. I refer to these debates as discourse, which I discuss next.

Discourse

I am using 'discourse' to mean the agreed or institutionalised way of talking, discussing or conversing about issues in a certain discipline, be they political, cultural or social. I see HIV and AIDS as a discipline with a discourse that has its own language and experts. Even as I argue that the discourse is surrounded by 'silence', this silence is selective as there are people who have 'learnt' the language, others have benefited financially from it, some have been silenced, while others have chosen to remain silent (as I discuss further in this chapter).

However, it is still a 'foreign' discourse especially as it is lacking a language that brings to light those painful and private experiences associated with the disease. It is worse when those affected are located in a class, culture and institutions (e.g., universities, as this study as others have shown) where space is not provided for private 'discourses'.

My reading of different feminist writings has clarified the meaning of discourse. One such feminist writer is Blackmore (1999) who defines discourses as:

> ...the institutionalised use of language, which can occur at a disciplinary, political, cultural and small group level...discourses

about women in leadership are informed by wider discourses about the politics of gender relations (p. 16).

Institutions, such as universities, are products of many different and often contradictory discourses and discursive fields. Kenway et al. (1994) enhance my understanding of discourse when they state that, "It is through discourse that meaning and human subjects are produced and through which power relations are maintained and changed" (p. 189). The questions that I have found central as I navigate the various discourses operating in universities and saw how women related to and were affected by them are:

- How is patriarchy functioning in the two universities and elsewhere?

- How is patriarchy produced, reproduced and regulated?

- What are the effects of patriarchy on women working in the two universities?

- How does patriarchy continue to exist (St. Pierre, 2000) (see the earlier on my understanding and use of the term patriarchy)?

St. Pierre (2000) argues that such questions can help one to:

...make patriarchy intelligible at the level of micro-practice, women can begin to make different statements about their lives...once women can locate and name the discourses and practices of patriarchy, they can begin to refuse them (p. 486).

Such an understanding of the HIV and AIDS discourse has assisted me in developing a language that can be useful in making transformative policies.

I have read the discourses operating in the interviews and discerned these truths that continue to maintain patriarchy in universities. Analysing the data from this study has given me a clear understanding of the different discursive fields and patriarchal structures and systems existing in the two universities. These are discussed further in Chapters Six to Ten, where the data is presented and discussed.

'The personal as political'

This phrase 'the personal is the political' was coined to draw attention to the political meanings of women's everyday experiences of their personal and private lives (Hughes, 2002). One definition of the phrase that I have found useful is provided by MacKinnon (1997):

> It means that women's distinctive experience as women occurs within that sphere that has been socially lived as the personal – private, emotional, interiorised, particular, individuated, intimate – so that what it is to know the politics of women's situations, is to know women's personal lives... (1997: 73).

In much feminist writing (e.g., Coate, 1999; Crosby, 1992; Edwards and Ribbens, 1998; Gold et al., 2002; Greed, 1990; hooks, 1994; Lewis, 1993; Mackinnon, 1997; Oakley, 2002; Stanley and Wise, 1983; Thomas, 1993), it has been argued that women feel silenced when bringing their personal experiences to the public even "where such 'personal' is the substance of what happens to us in the political" (Lewis, 1993: 3). The women's experiences that I listened to in this study were mainly occurring in their personal lives and they could be seen as 'private, particular and individuated'. Knowing women's lives as MacKinnon (1997) has noted is crucial in understanding women's situations.

Feminists have interrogated the gender boundaries between the personal and the political. Holmes (2000), for example, points out that those definitions of what is personal tend to associate it closely with the private and/or the domestic spheres and all that is supposed to belong within it. From this association of the personal with the private domain, Holmes (2000) notes that:

> Women, bodies, emotions and intimate relationships have been separated from the political world. Politics is defined as public, objective and rational – all qualities usually associated with masculinity. The public political sphere has been traditionally where men made decisions about what is 'the common good' (p. 305-306).

During the second wave of feminism, the slogan 'the personal is political' was coined (Holmes, 2000) and feminists rejected the traditional binary between the personal and the public.

There have been different meanings associated with this slogan. However, many feminists agree that the private/public division continues to be used to exclude differences and is, therefore, an issue in women's subordination.

Holmes (2000) claims that feminism as politics reclaims the personal domain by bringing it into public consideration and into the sphere of justice and public decision-making. By bringing women's private/personal experiences with HIV and AIDS into the public, I am asserting that their universities' responses to the pandemic need to take these experiences into account.

In Chapter Seven, I argue that the 'personal' can become 'political' if the social structures and systems of the two universities under study can change to become more accommodating and attentive to women's experiences. Any approaches that institutions might make in their responses to HIV and AIDS, which do not pay attention to aspects of gender integration, can remain on paper only, and will do little to tackle what is now commonly referred to as the third pandemic of stigma, which kills more than AIDS itself (Parker and Aggleton, 2003). On the need to integrate gender, Gupta et al. (2003) observe that:

> To fully integrate a gender perspective into all programming within an institution requires institutional systems, processes, and structures that routinely, continuously and comprehensively identify and respond appropriately to the different ways that gender affects programming (p. 26).

A gendered approach, therefore, requires a change in the systems and the total processes of the way a system is run. Universities have been noted to have structures that are basically women-unfriendly (Morley, 2003b); hence, there is need to change this if gender is to be integrated in any programmes and policies.

Care is another concept that this study has shown to fall in the private domain, yet it has an impact on the public roles of women. In the following section, I discuss how the concept of care is used in this study while relating it to the issue of making the personal political.

Care

One of the main gender issues in HIV and AIDS is that of caring for people living with the disease (Kelly, 2003). The women in my study talked about their caring responsibilities when people close to them were sick and the varying effects these responsibilities had on them.

Hughes (2002) notes that, although there is a diversity of meanings, indicators and variables associated with care, there has been some consistency in the way feminists have analysed this term. Research in the area of care-giving has shown that women are the ones who perform the role and are perceived to be mainly responsible for the physical and emotional work of care-giving (e.g., Boyd, 2002; Delphy and Leonard, 1992; Duongsaa, 2004; Henry, 1996; Marcus, 1993; McKie et al., 2001; Miroiu, 2003; Olenja, 1999; Outshoorn, 2002; Thomas, 1993). It is notable that care work, especially that which is not paid for or valued seems to be done predominantly by women. This cuts across many nations and cultures as suggested in the literature from different regions of the world (Boyd, 2002; Coleman, 2002; Delphy and Leonard, 1992; Hatt et al., 1999; Henry, 1996; Hughes, et al., 2005; Hughes, 2002; Jones and Rupp, 2000; Marcus, 1993; Olenja, 1999; Romanin and Over, 1993; Wickham-Searl, 1992).

In the context of HIV and AIDS, women are likely to be looking after the sick in the homes, taking them to hospitals, making sure that patients have taken their drugs, cleaning and cooking for them. Women's care work, which is mainly free and voluntary, goes unnoticed and is hardly considered as work in the field of policy and programming (Olenja, 1999).

The interconnection between women's career progression and their gender roles has been noted in feminist research. In one such research reported by Deem (2003), 137 male and female manager-academics (from Heads of Department to Vice Chancellors) in 16 universities in the UK were interviewed. The careers of female and male manager–academics were analysed to see if gender power relations, expectations and discrimination had affected their careers and organisational experiences.

This study also examined whether and how gender relations and cultures were perceived to be relevant to management. The research findings suggested that women's participation in management roles, their perceptions about their practices and the expectations others held of them were still marked by gender (Deem, 2003). While few men in this study thought that their careers had been affected by their own gender, women were seen as disadvantaged by gender particularly motherhood. Fatherhood was not seen to harm men's academic careers.

Although the women that my study targeted said they usually employed domestic help, this did not always mean that women are completely free of domestic work and other gender roles. Delphy and Leonard (2002) argue that:

> Having servants in itself involves work for women. Servants have to be hired, trained and managed (management and training in industry are not usually seen as idleness). They also require emotional work; helpers have to be listened to, praised, made to feel important, and to have their anxieties soothed, etc (p.178).

In addition to the usual domestic chores that Kenyan professional women have become accustomed to, AIDS has presented new challenges and responsibilities of caring for sick members of their immediate families and distant relatives. Many of those employed to work in the homes are hesitant to look after sick people, especially those suffering from AIDS because of stigma and the fear that they may become infected. There is a need to look into the new responsibilities facing professional women in the context of HIV and AIDS and have it considered in policy formulation as child care has been considered in a country like the Netherlands (Outshoorn, 2002).

I carried out the present study while aware of the differences that exist among senior university women about societal expectations to provide care, especially for relatives Differences such as age, marital status, socio-economic status, religious affiliation and ethnicity were taken into consideration during the selection of women interviewees. I had a fair representation of all these categories as shown in the profile of participants shown in Table 1. The findings of this study however have indicated that there were no differences in care giving responsibilities of the women from the different categories as I show in Chapter Seven.

Demands on women to provide care appear fairly universal, and indeed many women make conscious decisions to care for others. Much debate still continues among feminists (e.g., Adkins, 2002; Cockburn, 2002; Hochschild, 2002) about introducing workplace policies that recognise the private aspects of employees, especially women. To make a case for women's private needs and issues which need to be factored in workplace policies, especially in this time of rising AIDS cases, I support some of the arguments of radical feminists. For example, I agree with Alsop, Fitzsimons and Lemon (2002) who argue that some women's characteristics need to be a cause for celebration rather than condemnation.

There may not be a consensus about what women's characteristics are. In this study they appear to be caring, emotional understanding, support and sensuality. The role of caring that women provide to others in the HIV and AIDS era is to be celebrated not ignored or degraded. Many women can continue with their roles as long as they are recognised and rewarded accordingly. The other challenge is that these roles would only be factored into the policy and practice of institutions if they are talked about or made public, an issue that I discuss next.

Silence

Clinton (2003 p. 369) has observed that too many women, in too many countries, speak the same language of silence. In Chapters One and Two, I have argued that educated and well-off Kenyan women have been silenced by the current debates about HIV and AIDS in Africa, which have continued to focus on behaviour models. I use silence in this study to mean that those issues, especially concerning women, are unspoken, taken for granted, or seen as though they cannot be challenged. Such issues are ignored because it is believed that that is the way they should be – mainly because they favour men – in a patriarchal system that characterises social functioning in Kenya. Women themselves may choose to remain silent for fear of the consequences if they talk, or for lack of a channel through which they can talk, or simply feeling that it is better to live with the status quo than to challenge it.

Silence emerges as an important issue in this study and other related studies that I have reviewed (e.g., Acker, 1994; Caplan, 1993; Gold, 1995; Gold et al., 2002; hooks, 1994; Humpreys and Gutenby, 1999; Luke, 1994; McFadden, 2003; Miller, 1998; Morley, 1999, 2003b). On African women's silencing, Kolawole (1997) argues that they were vocal in "orature but silent in literature" (p. 4). Kolawole (1997) further notes that African women have always had their voice although in different forms from modern types of 'voice', which are connected with public voice.

The discourse of silence has some contrasts because people who may not consider themselves as silenced, like university women, may indeed be silenced in ways that they may not even be aware of. In some cases, women may want to be silent about private matters (Luke, 1994) especially if there is no safe place in which to express themselves. Similarly, hooks (1994) argues that silence is connected to whose voice has authority, which is related to class, race, gender and knowledge.

One's class, race, gender and knowledge can contribute to them being silenced, or having a voice or even choosing to remain silent. Those who choose to remain silent may do so because of feeling 'othered' from the discourse, or if the discourse is viewed as 'foreign'. Gold (1995), for example, notes that women can be, and have been, silenced especially when they enter into a foreign discourse. I see the discourse of HIV and AIDS in relation to women in universities as a 'foreign discourse' or what Gold (1995: 111) refers to as 'the impenetrable discourse' in ways that I briefly discuss here.

The fact that HIV and AIDS have been persistently linked with sexuality, promiscuity, poverty and death has led to a 'deafening silence' around the discourse, not just in Kenya but in the international arena, as noted in the literature (Barnett and Whiteside, 2002; Baylies and Bujra 2000; Hunter, 2003; Kaleeba and Ray, 1997; Preece and Ntseane, 2004; Roth and Hogan, 1998; Sabatier, 1988; Smith, 2002; Treichler and Warren, 1998; Vliet, 1996). For senior women in higher education, there is a double silence as far as HIV and AIDS is concerned. The first silence is linked to the nature of universities, which, as documented by a great deal of feminist research, are not receptive or 'attentive' to the experiences of women and other less powerful groups (Anderson and Williams, 2001; Bagilhoe, 1994; Deem, 2003; Gold et al., 2002; hooks, 1994; Lewis, 1993; Lund, 1998; Morley, 1999, 2000, 2003b; Morley and Walsh, 1996; Onsongo, 2000; Probert, 2005; Romanin and Over, 1993; Singh, 2003;Smith, 2002).

It has also been documented that many African universities have been 'silent' about the impact of HIV and AIDS on senior staff (ACU and DFID, 2001; Bollag, 2001; Chetty, 2000; Kelly, 2003b; Mullens, 2003; Nyutho et al., 2005; Nzioka, 2000; Otaala, 2000; Owino, 2004). This silence in universities can be viewed as a consequence of the ways in which HIV and AIDS education about prevention and care has been handled, both locally and internationally.

In the initial years of the epidemic, experiences of men served to define the disease so that women disappeared from the scene (Ankrah, 1996a, 1996b; Sherr et al., 1996). Later on, when women were 'seen', it was in the context of blame (Baylies, 2000). Attention was focused on so-called 'risky groups' of people, among them commercial sex workers, poor populations in the slums and generally those considered to be promiscuous (Campbell, 2003; VSO, 2003). This focus on those seen to be at 'risk' obscured the increasing 'risk' among those generally viewed as safe (Campbell, 2003).

The women targeted by my research would normally be viewed as safe from HIV infection by many of the behaviour models that have been used in HIV and AIDS research (VSO, 2003) as they do not fit the above stereotypes of those at risk. They are thus invisible or are silenced. This silencing is noted by Chetty (2000) when he points out the discomfort surrounding the disclosure of HIV status by people of high social status, especially those in the higher education community. The silence does not only affect those infected, but also those affected.

It becomes increasingly difficult to even talk about experiences about family members infected by HIV and AIDS. This is because such disclosure seems to make people question the morality of one's family members, an issue that was raised by one of the women in this study (see Chapter Seven). On AIDS-related silence, denial and stigma,

Parker and Aggleton (2003) argue that this has continued to be a global issue. A feminist theoretical framework, therefore, has provided me with a constructive discourse to analyse these silences, stigma and denial (see Chapter Nine). Feminist theory gives some visibility and legitimacy to women's experiences not just with regard to HIV and AIDS, but also other personal challenges that women may experience in different ways from men (see Chapter Seven).

While some African feminists have condemned African women's silences (e.g., McFadden, 2003; Thiam, 1986) others like Pereira (2003) argue that instead of condemning the silences, it would be more productive to map them with a view to their further exploration and understanding. Pereira (2003) particularly picks on silences around sexuality (see Chapter Nine), which she notes have many causes that need to be understood in terms of "what they are about, what noises are filling these silences, and how to transform those silences into more appropriate responses" (p. 62). Through the data presented in the chapters that follow, I have attempted to interpret the silences of the women that I interviewed in ways that Pereira (2003) has argued.

Summary and Conclusion

From my attempt to explain how feminist perspectives informed my study, I have noted the difficulty of one trying to identify with any particular strand of feminist theorising. In this chapter I have explained why I chose to work with a mixture of ideas informed by feminism without labelling my work as belonging to one stance or the other. I have outlined the concepts that have guided me from stating my research question, my data collection, my data analysis and, indeed, the writing process. The issues and concepts discussed in this chapter provide my study with a framework that helps me to link the themes that emerged from the interviews with theory. This has enabled me to look at the women's experiences beyond their situations, but as incidents that could be used to understand other women's experiences.

= 6

The Status of Women in the Sampled Universities

Dominant groups remain privileged because they write the rules, and the rules they write enable them to continue to write the rules

Reskin (2000: 257)

Introduction

The purpose of this chapter is to address the question: What is the status of women in the management of the two universities in the study and how can their positions explain their silences and invisibilities in relation to university AIDS policies and programmes?

Universities have been singled out as places where women continue to be under-represented in senior academic and administrative positions (Mabokela, 2003). I wanted to gain insights into women's experiences in the two universities. I hope that these insights will inform the process of creating institutional environments that are supportive of women's professional endeavours. I believe that knowledge about women's career experiences would especially be helpful in informing HIV and AIDS policies and programmes in the two universities.

In Chapter Two, I noted that Kenyan women are faced with many challenges, which often keep them in lower ranks in the workplace. In this chapter, I use the findings of this study to show the gender disparities that exist in Weruini and Holy Ghost Universities.

This is followed by a discussion on the barriers that women in this study pointed out as hindering their career progression. My aim is to show that the under-representation of women in senior positions, coupled with failure by the two universities to recognise the need for policies and practices that can protect women's rights, increases women's invisibility when faced with challenges like those presented by HIV and AIDS.

The chapter comprises the following:

- A brief overview of the status of women in universities globally and how this is reflected in Kenya;

- Some sex disaggregated gender segregated data of seven most senior academic and administrative positions that are comparable in Weruini and Holy Ghost Universities; and,

- A discussion of factors seen to contribute to the lower status of women compared to men (they include cultural/gender stereotypes, women's career experiences, limited access to doctoral studies, and lack of support for women's research).

A Brief Overview of Women's Status in Universities Globally and in Kenya

The under-representation of women in the academic and administrative hierarchies of universities has been a concern for many feminist researchers as demonstrated by the amount of literature available (Ankrah, 1996b; Coate, 1999; Currie et al.; 2002; Grunberg, 2001; Hall, 1996; Kearney, 2000; Lund, 1998; Mabokela, 2003; Morley and Walsh, 1996; Onsongo, 2005). Research about the status of women in Kenyan universities continues to show that women hardly rise to senior positions both in academics and administration (Kamau, 2002; Kanake, 1995; Khasiani, 2000; Manya, 2000; Onsongo, 2005). One would expect universities to have norms associated with gender equity, which would afford women equal opportunities for academic advancement.

On this lack of gender equity in universities, Acker (1994) observes that academic life is one area where, in theory, women would find few barriers to opportunity and it is in universities where women could have successful careers. However, this is not always the case as Acker (1994) notes:

> What needs to be explained is why we find women academics so relatively disadvantaged and men so firmly in control. Why we have a man-centred university with some women in it (p. 137).

Research into higher education has suggested that in order for academics to rise to seniority, they not only need to teach, but they also need to carry out research, publish and present their work in conferences (Bagilhoe, 1994; Khasiani, 2000; Kwesiga, 2002; Mabokela, 2003; Miroiu, 2003; Morley, 1999; Morley and Walsh, 1996; Onsongo, 2000, 2005; Probert, 2005; Singh, 2002). However, these studies suggest that even when women meet these criteria, often set by men (because of their majority in the decision-making bodies), women hardly manage the break through the 'glass ceiling.'

While socio-cultural conditions facing female academics differ significantly in different countries, their experiences are remarkably similar. Further analysis of universities has indicated that institutional policies and women's personal and domestic challenges contribute to their remaining in lower ranks compared to men (Anderson andWilliams, 2001; Brooks and Mackinnon, 2001; Kamau, 2002; Mabokela, 2003; Morley, 1999, 2003b; Onsongo, 2005).

As I have noted in Chapters One and Two, HIV and AIDS have presented a new set of challenges for Kenyan women, especially the educated and economically well-to-do who are not usually associated with this pandemic. These challenges have made women's struggle to survive on equal terms with men in higher education even harder and more complicated (Garland, 2001; see also Chapter Seven).

Senior university women in Kenya would be considered to be well-off economically than the majority in the country. Many of them live in towns where hospitals are easily accessible resulting in relatives who require medical attention to seek accommodation in these women's homes (see Chapter Two). This has meant that many women working in universities are finding themselves being called upon to look after their sick relatives, to take care of orphaned children, and to pay medical bills among other obligations. This situation adds extra responsibilities to the tasks of these women who are already burdened by the challenges that university careers present as noted in the literature (Grunberg, 2001; Mabokela, 2003; Morley, 1999, 2003a, 2003b; Morley et al., 2005; Morley and Walsh, 1996; Onsongo, 2000; Wyn et al., 2000).

In the current era of HIV and AIDS, Kenyan women need to overcome various hurdles in order to survive on an equal basis with men in universities. To illustrate the extent of the inequalities that exist, the next section focuses on the status of women in Holy Ghost and Weruini Universities at the time of this study.

Senior Positions by Gender at Holy Ghost and Weruini

Information about the positions women hold in universities is crucial when one wants to improve the gender imbalance (Lund, 1998). Collecting gender segregated data can be difficult because much of the statistics are not gender specific. In this study, for example, I had hoped to gather data for positions from assistant lecturer and above. I discovered that the records available only listed total numbers without gender specification. Where names were used, say in the case of department heads, it was difficult to tell if it was male or female. It is for this reason that I worked with the top positions where I could easily confirm the gender. The data is presented in Table 3.

The above data shows the existing gender inequalities at the senior academic and management positions in the two universities. It is only the post of Head Librarian, which tends to be occupied by women in both universities. It would appear that women are commonly employed as librarians at universities anywhere (Singh, 2003).

Table 3: Senior faculty and administrative positions by gender

Position	Weruini	Holy Ghost	Male	Female
Vice Chancellor	1	-	1	-
Deputy Vice Chancellor	2	1	2	-
Full Professor	18	6	2	-
Associate Professor	18	6	1	1
Head Librarian	1	1	-	-
Registrar	2	1	1	-
Deans	4	2	3	1

At the time of this study, none of the six Kenyan public universities had a woman Vice Chancellor and only two out of 19 of the private ones had women VCs. This changed in April 2006, when the first woman was appointed Vice Chancellor of one of the public universities.

Vice Chancellors of public universities used to be presidential appointees. In 2003, there was a change of government and the universities were given powers by the President to hire VCs through a competitive selection process. Kenyatta University was the first one to appoint a woman VC through a competitive recruitment. This is an indication that changing the hiring and promotion rules can help to open doors for more women into senior management positions (Manya, 2000).

Chancellors of the public universities are still appointed by the President. In 2003, the President appointed Chancellors for all the six public universities, but no woman was appointed. This is likely to change if the selection of Chancellors is also made competitive like that of the Vice Chancellors, hence making it possible for more women to move into these senior positions.

Scarcity of women within the academic hierarchy has been said to hinder the women's ability to influence the policy and direction of their institutions (Kearney, 2000). In Wyn et al.'s (2000) study of Australian and Canadian women managers, the senior women saw their positions in terms of making a difference to others. These women were said to have seen this difference in areas of "equity, democracy, anti-sexism, anti-racism and participation" (Wyn et al., 2000: 442). However, all the women in this study viewed themselves as feminists.

Women who are not feminists may not necessarily work towards changes that may benefit other women and disadvantaged groups, as has been noted by Onsongo in Kenya (2005) and Morley in Europe (1999). Even feminists may go through what Morley refers to as "a process of masculinisation" (p. 75). One woman in Wyn et al.' s (2000) study expressed this 'masculinisation' when she noted that there were ways in which she had learnt to do things in the traditional ways. This woman said that at times she did not always work for radical change. She found institutional practices already in place easier to use than to challenge. Similarly, Mabokela (2003) notes that due to the small representation of women in predominantly male organisations, they may be subjected to treatment that compromises the contributions they could make in their organisations.

In addition to the above arguments, my conversations with several women after recorded interviews (as noted in my field notes) indicated that if more awareness is created about the factors that hinder women's progression, then some women could challenge them if in positions to do so (see also Chapter Eight). My intention in having informal talk-sessions after the interviews was to provide the women with a chance to further reflect on the issues we had discussed in the interview. It is through these reflections that the women seemed to be more aware of some of the hindrances they had faced in their careers, and had not thought about them as caused by patriarchy in their institutions. Dr. Wangare, for example, went to great lengths to discuss with me the challenges she had faced when trying to get her PhD scholarship. She said that she would want to see her department set up a women's network, which could help younger women academics to access scholarships. This reflexivity, I hoped, would help them to want to 'make a difference' if they were in a position to do so.

Some of the women had already done this as noted by one of the respondents:

A few years ago, I was at the forefront of a group of women who wanted a sexual harassment policy in the institution. Initially, when we presented our ideas, the issue was brushed off. We decided the best thing was to form a group.... We used to meet once a month ... It was during these meetings that we discussed issues affecting us as women and we decided to go to the VC. We discussed sexual harassment and lack of security on campus because there were no lights ... We wrote a concept paper and the VC funded a workshop where we invited the CEO of the Forum for African Women Educationalists (FAWE) and we deliberated on all these things. The workshop recommended that adequate lighting be provided on campus and measures on sexual harassment to be put in place. Security lights were fitted, but unfortunately, the woman who was selected to write the policy on sexual harassment was not committed and the whole thing died out. That VC left and we are yet to approach the new one...but working as a group made the VC to listen... I think this is one of the ways women should work together in universities on issues such as AIDS (Dr Kaiga, Lecturer, Weruini).

One of the issues raised by Dr. Kaiga is that when women who are committed to change work together, then some achievements can be realised. In their case, they were able to have lights fitted in campus. However, as noted earlier in this chapter, it would be wrong to assume that all women would be committed to change that would be favourable to them. From this example given by Dr. Kaiga, the woman who was appointed by the VC to lead in drafting a sexual harassment policy failed to do so and the initiative died. Thus, as Morley (1999) observes:

...the presence of women in senior positions is not an accurate measure of organisational development, as female cannot be unilaterally equated with feminism, nor are all feminists reflexive about their location in organisational power relations (p. 75).

Even with the differing views about what women can or cannot do when in positions of leadership, I agree with Deem's (2003) conclusion that, "without more women in senior-manager academic posts, it is unlikely that some kinds of alternative approaches explored in the literature on women managers will develop' (p. 255). It is for this reason that I explore factors that hinder more women from attaining senior manager and academic posts in the two universities.

Gender stereotypes

One of the factors implied by the women as an impediment to their careers was that of stereotypes. These are beliefs about what men and women can or cannot do simply because of their gender. The common stereotypes about women brand them as unstable and emotional, characteristics that are not suitable for managers (Ouston, 1993). The construction of gendered expectations, beliefs and stereotypes does not usually begin in the workplace. It begins beyond work, school and even beyond national boundaries. The discourse surrounding boys' and girls' differences and identities resonates in internationally recommended textbooks, in the leadership that is mostly male dominated, in the people who hold and get different types of jobs, and in media images. Generally, Kenyan women are perceived as incapable of coping with management positions and this perception discourages many of them from aspiring to become managers (Khamisi, 2005; Odhiambo, 2005).

Women tend to have difficulty in developing an authoritative voice, and they may be modest about their own achievements and knowledge (Aisenberg and Harrington, 1988). Making a reputation in the academy and in all workplaces requires self-advertisement, which may not always be easy for women (Mabokela, 2003). Research continues to suggest that characteristics for success tend to be stereotyped as masculine and women have problems coping with a mainly male peer group and its expectations of them to be like men (Onsongo, 2005; Reskin, 2000; Wyn et al., 2000).

On the need for women to market themselves in the university, Mabokela's (2003) study of South African women academics found that women are "socialised to diminish their accomplishments and their achievements, as a way of being feminine"(p. 143). Academic careers may not be seen as feminine as noted by one woman in my study:

> When a woman decides to enter the profession of men, it is not always easy. Lecturers are supposed to be men, not single young women! You are considered an outcast and a disgrace if you are seen challenging and threatening men. Some colleagues look at me suspiciously, but even students seem to think I am not qualified enough to be their teacher. I have heard them asking 'is she a lecturer?' I try very hard to prove to them that being young and a woman does not make me any less qualified, but I can assure you some of these stereotypes can discourage some people (Ms Mueni, Lecturer, Holy Ghost University).

As I pointed out in Chapter Two, the Kenyan society is generally unsupportive of women's career progression. Women are not usually encouraged to aspire for senior positions and especially not in 'masculine' careers like university teaching (Maathai, 2006). There is a silent fear that if a woman becomes very senior she risks not getting a husband, yet marriage is held in very high regard in Kenya (Kuria, 2003; Machera, 2004). This is not unique to Kenya as Reskin (2000) raises similar issues about women professionals in the United States.

Gaining the required postgraduate qualifications for university teaching, also presents challenges to women, an issue I return to in later in the present chapter. Some women, even when they have a chance to further their studies, may fear that being 'overeducated' might reduce their chances of finding husbands. Because of the way men and women are socialised in Kenya, a woman is generally expected to achieve less than her husband both in education and career progression (Maathai, 2006). In effect, fewer women than men opt for further studies. This is one factor that could lead to having a small number of senior women in universities.

Ms Mueni, a young unmarried woman, whom I have quoted above, said that her potential suitors seem to become discouraged when they learn she is a university lecturer. In an earlier study I carried out in a private university in Kenya, a single woman told me how she had delayed going for further studies because she was hoping to get married before taking up her PhD studies to avoid limiting her chances of getting a husband (Kamau, 2001). I met this woman four years later, and learnt that she had been married. She was at the time looking for a scholarship to pursue her doctoral studies. She was by then already past 40 years of age, hence her chances of completing her studies, combined with the challenges of a young family, could mean she may be already too late to rise to the professor level (see also Chapter Six). Similar experiences were shared by women interviewed by Onsongo (2005).

Gender stereotypes can discourage some women from aspiring to develop themselves even when they have the opportunities, as one of my interviewees told me. She said that her male and female colleagues made some negative comments when she told them she had been awarded a scholarship to study in the UK:

> When I learnt that I had been given the scholarship, I came here and told my colleagues. I heard from them things that were only making me get discouraged. They would say 'Hey, how can you leave your children, there is nothing that would make me leave my children.' Those things really mixed me up. I started asking myself, 'Am I doing the right thing?' One man asked me 'Hey, you are going because you have no husband, if it were my wife, she could not go'. I decided to challenge him by asking, 'If it were you who was going, could your wife stop you from going?' He said, 'No but if she is the one I wouldn't, you are going because you are not answerable to anybody'. So I stopped talking to people at Weruini and that is when the depression decreased (Dr. Wangare, Senior Lecturer, Weruini).

Dr. Wangare's experience reveals contradictions and complex processes available in women's careers. This complexity is expressed by Wyn et al. (2000) when they note that a single event like a promotion in a woman's life may be both "positive and negative, welcome and problematic, inclusive and marginalising" (p. 438). In Dr. Wangare's case, getting a scholarship became a source of ridicule for her. She described the reactions of her colleagues as depressing. Yet she had struggled a lot to get this scholarship (see further in this chapter). Such reactions could make some women give up on their opportunities altogether.

Closely related to gender stereotypes, women may also face other personal challenges that affect their career choices. Dr. Wangare, for example, narrated the struggles she underwent trying to place her children in boarding schools. This was made more difficult by the fact that she had a very short notice to report for her studies. Being divorced may have helped Wangare because she did not need to seek permission from a husband (see her comments earlier in this chapter). However, things may have been a lot easier if the husband was available and willing to stay with the children. In her case, the children had to change schools; she also had to vacate her house and move all her belongings to her mother's house. She however told me that her women friends offered invaluable help.

In addition to challenges presented by children and other more familiar commitments that affect women, HIV and AIDS has created new challenges that have had an effect on women's careers as I show in Chapters Seven and Eight.

Domestic Challenges and Women's Careers

Studies from different parts of the world suggest that women's social obligations may have a negative impact on their career progression (Blackmore, 1999; Coleman, 2002 in the UK; Moore, 1999 in Israel; Morley, 1999 in Europe; Romanin and Over, 1993 in Australia). In Romanin and Over's study (1993), men and women who held a full-time appointment at lecturer level and above in Australian universities in 1988 were compared in terms of the career paths they followed, geographic mobility, domestic responsibilities, work roles and levels of performance as academics. The women in this study had more often spent a period outside the workforce or in part-time employment due to child-care responsibilities.

The findings of this survey showed that there were more women than men combining full-time work and household labour. However, even when numbers of children and their ages were considered, there were no differences between men and women in self-rated performance in such academic roles as teaching, research and administration. The responsibilities that women have outside work contribute to attitudes of male managers which brand women as lazy or uncommitted to academic life (Kamau, 2002). Such attitudes can influence decisions about recruitment and promotion (Onsongo, 2005).

Many Kenyan career women give first priority to their families, not because they lack commitment to their jobs, but because they have been socialised that a good woman thinks of her family first (Kanake, 1995; Maathai, 2006; Onsongo, 2005). These are sentiments that were raised by many of the women after the interviews, which I noted in my field diary. Many of them argued that a woman rarely feels complete unless her family has been successful. Mrs Wandera, for example, noted that she would rather give up on her PhD than fail to prepare good meals for her family and support her husband, who she noted was a very busy man (from field notes).

Before this 'script' of socialisation is changed, it would be useful if institutions took into account gender roles, especially when planning for issues like staff development. For example, scholarships to study abroad would benefit more women if such scholarships can support whole families, especially in cases of women with young children. One of the women I interviewed spoke about how earlier in her career she had declined a British Council scholarship, which had required her to leave Kenya to study in Britain. She did not think that her decision affected her career progression. She said she got another job later as a librarian and received another scholarship to study locally. However, as she confesses below, the reasons for not taking the first scholarship were driven by her social responsibilities as a woman:

> When I was much younger, I got a scholarship shortly after I had found a job in Nairobi where my husband was, as I had been working

upcountry. I declined to take the scholarship for two reasons. One, I did not think it would be a good idea to separate the family again. Two, my son was three years old and I felt that was not a good time to leave him (Mrs Mwithaga, Librarian, Holy Ghost University).

Morley (1999) observes that it is difficult for many women to follow age-related linear career paths because of issues like the ones Mrs Mwithaga talked about. In a study of career paths of women academics in Australia, Probert (2005) found that the significant differences between men and women's experiences lie in their living responsibilities. Men were much less likely to have partners in full-time employment. In her focus groups, which involved 15 women, Probert (2005) found that a number had broken up with their partners when completing their doctorates. This increased the caring responsibilities (which included care for adolescent children and elderly parents) for the women interviewed.

Probert (2005) notes that the above are issues that are not dealt with in normal 'family-friendly' policies in institutions. An example of family-friendly policy is whereby scholarships for staff development provide family packages. Many scholarships target younger people who are less than 35 years, a time when many women have young children. Such factors may also lead to the disparities seen at senior levels as many women may lose out on opportunities for professional development early in their careers.

Besides the domestic responsibilities that either keep women in the bottom ranks or are used as an excuse not to promote them, there are other discriminatory practices in universities. Some are explicit and others implicit, but they continue to keep women in the low positions of their institutions. An example is limited access to doctoral studies for women as I discuss next.

Challenges with Doctoral Studies

One area where Kenyan university women face subtle discrimination is that of further studies, especially when attempting to pursue doctorates (Kamau, 2001; Onsongo, 2000, 2005). Discrimination is not always easy to define. It can be direct or indirect and it can manifest itself in individual behaviour or in institutional practices. Some discrimination can be legislated against, while other forms of discrimination of an attitudinal or behavioural nature are more difficult to identify and eradicate (Anderson and Williams, 2001). I will focus on the attitudinal discrimination, which women may not be aware of, hence making it difficult to fight against.

There are some rules and regulations in universities, which indirectly discriminate against women, yet initially they appear neutral. Thus, many times women are unaware of the biased rules, leading to silence about the issue. It is usually men who make many university rules and regulations, while promotion and selection procedures are geared to a stereotypical image of a male leader (Brooks and Mackinnon, 2001; Kearney, 2000; Ruijs, 1993).

Some of the discriminatory attitudes that women face in the university can become a source of low motivation and may have an effect on their career progression (Onsongo, 2005). Attaining a doctorate remains a prerequisite to attaining higher status in universities (Probert, 2005). However, as the women in this study told me, there are several limitations that continue to stop them from taking up or even completing their PhDs.

In Kenya, not many women hold doctorates (Kamau, 2001; Khasiani, 2000), yet many universities still require a PhD as the minimum qualification to join academia. Obtaining a doctorate for a woman in Kenya is usually much more challenging than it is for men, especially because the country does not have well-established doctoral programmes and those that exist are in limited fields (Kamau, 2001). Studying abroad remains one of the viable options for many academics. However, challenges related to the family can discourage women academics who wish to pursue doctoral studies abroad, an issue I have discussed in this chapter.

About this, Leonard (2001) notes that husbands also may not support the idea of their partners pursuing higher degrees and they can actually prove a bigger obstacle than children can. Leonard (2001) reckons that wives are more likely to support their husbands through the uphill struggle of completing a doctorate degree than husbands who may threaten, or even ask for a divorce. In Probert's (2005) study of women academics in Australia, it emerged that eight of the ten women had broken up with their partners while they were studying for their PhDs.

HIV and AIDS have increased the challenges for Kenyan women wishing to pursue doctorates both locally and abroad, an issue I discuss in Chapter Seven. Studying locally presents a new set of challenges to women as it usually means combining full-time teaching, family and community responsibilities with their studies. Negotiating for study leave, even when one has a scholarship is another gender issue, which is not always guaranteed as I learnt from some of the women in this study. The following is an extract of one woman who was taking a long distance PhD with the University of South Africa (UNISA) while still teaching:

> I have been writing my PhD proposal for the last year...for some months now, I have not had a house help... I was tempted to just forget the housework and complete my proposal but I felt no, I have to cook nice food for my husband and children.... We also have a farm, which I have to look after as my husband can't go because he is a deputy principal so he leaves everything to me...The university work is also overwhelming...Like now, I have a lot of marking and the students want feedback ... Unless I get funding to spend at least two months in South Africa where I can complete the proposal and come back to do the research, then it might take many years to complete the studies – yet I am an old woman. At the moment HG can only pay for my ticket and a stay of two weeks so I need to have completed the proposal because two weeks is too short and I need to receive feedback from my supervisors. I feel like giving up but talking to you has also encouraged me to continue (Mrs Wandera, Lecturer, Holy Ghost University).

Mrs Wandera was 56 years old at the time of this study. She struck me as a hard working and determined woman. As her experiences show, even at her age, it was still difficult to combine studying, work and family. She said that her husband was supportive of her career; however, due to his very demanding position as a deputy principal of a fairly large college, all the household responsibilities are left to her. Deem (2003) documents similar findings where unequal household divisions of labour were recognised as important by a majority of women respondents in respect of academic careers. Only a few of male respondents in Deem's study thought that their careers had been affected by their gender. Judging from her age and the time it may take her to complete her PhD Mrs Wandera is not likely to be promoted to the next rank of senior lecturer by the time she retires.

Mrs Wandera's experiences are not isolated, as similar findings are documented by Probert (2005) in an Australian survey. In Probert's survey, 12.2 per cent of women and 32.8 per cent of men held a PhD at the time of their first appointment to universities. The study also revealed that among those who began their careers without a PhD, women were less likely to go on and complete one than men.

Many of the women in my study said they had problems with funding for their doctoral studies. University and government funds are surrounded by too much micro-politics and bureaucracy, which generally works to the disadvantage of women, as Dr. Wangare's experience shows below:

> There were forms for commonwealth scholarships for PhD, which are usually given to government institutions. On learning about their availability at the university, I asked my dean to give me one. The dean told me he had only one copy...I went to the registrar academic who told me the forms were finished ... So I went to the British Council and they gave me one...I did not send the form through the university as I feared the dean may not forward them so I just sent them straight to the university... I was admitted without funding ... I needed to raise the funds ... I went to 'A' Trust who gave me 1,000 sterling pounds per year for three years. I went to 'B' and they gave me 5,000 pounds per year; so I had 6,000 pounds, but I needed 14,000 per year. After a year 'A' withdrew their funding, as I had not yet claimed it. I was worried I could also lose the 'B' money as well.... So I continued searching ...One day I got a letter from the university that

had admitted me instructing me to report in a month's time. They had decided to give me the balance... My dear, it was unbelievable! ...I put my children in boarding schools and left without study leave which I was denied as the university claimed that I had not gone through them to get the scholarship so they had nothing to do with it. A year later, they wrote to me and gave me three years paid leave (Dr. Wangare, Senior Lecturer, Weruini).

Dr. Wangare's experiences suggest that various discriminatory practices exist, which especially affect women. Many of those in charge are likely to be male as was the case with Dr. Wangare where both the dean and the registrar just wanted to frustrate her. Practices of frustrating women who try to pursue further studies or even seek promotion have been reported in other studies (Kamau, 2001; Onsongo, 2005).

In order for women to make it to senior positions, they may require determination, patience and lack of fear of becoming unpopular amongst colleagues. Sometimes when women portray such qualities, they may be seen as aggressive, a trait that can be used against them (Wyn et al., 2000). Research on women's issues could help reveal the problems they face and provide a basis to challenge them. A lack of institutional support for such research also emerged as contributing to invisibility of women's issues as I discuss in the following section.

Lack of Support for Women's Research

Some feminist researchers (Acker et al., 1991; Mabokela, 2003; Onsongo, 2005;Wyn et al., 2000) have noted that universities are not always supportive of research on women, especially if it is termed 'feminist'. In their study on women Wyn et al. (2000) note that:

> In some cases, their areas of research were seen to be marginal to the central 'mainstream' concerns of education... for others, discriminatory practices by heads of departments and in some cases deans, were aimed at holding them back' (p. 493).

Regular gender audits are especially helpful as they form a basis for affirmative action (Mabokela, 2003). Feminist or women's research also helps to create awareness for both men and women about issues normally taken for granted.

According to Barnes (2005), research done by African women scholars has mainly received support from donors, outside of universities. Barnes (2005), for example, notes that the lack of support for women's research from within the universities implies that:

> Work of women academics and 'gender work' remain viable as intellectual production, but dependent in some large measure on donor funds, and on activities, which only occur outside the ambit of institutionally demarcated boundaries. Women academics are therefore working harder, differently, and in riskier environments (in terms of sustainability) – to maintain and increase their intellectual production (p. 9).

In Kenya, Onsongo (2005) observes that research, which is termed 'feminist', may not be taken as seriously as other forms of research. Hence, as Barnes (2005) notes, sustainability of research by women, and especially on women's issues, is threatened as universities rarely fund such research.

My experience during the pilot to this study also showed that feminist research is misunderstood and not taken seriously. Before I left London for Kenya, I had contacted a male dean in a public university and informed him that I intended to go to his university for the pilot study. I told him that I was looking at whether his university's responses to HIV and AIDS were gender-sensitive. When I later went to his office, he commented that since I was interested in women's issues, he would not know who else could help me apart from the women at the Gender Institute. He introduced me to the Acting Director of the Institute. I had hoped that I would interview this man in his capacity as a dean. However, he made it clear that he would not be interested in 'those women's and feminist things... please talk to the other women in the Gender Institute' (Pilot study field notes April 5, 2004).

As Deem (2003) notes, "Gender in this sense still equates to women" (p. 255). I realised that in order to access male and female respondents and for my work to be taken seriously, it was necessary that I did not mention its feminist or gender nature. I considered this as ethical and justified because through this kind of research, women's issues can be known and hopefully acted on. Such a study also helps to develop knowledge to show what actually happens in women's daily world and how these events are experienced (Probert, 2005).

I realised (as I noted in my field notes) that the women in this study may not consider themselves feminists. Many of them may not have gone through a similar feminist journey like the one I have undergone (see Chapter Five). Only one interviewee, Dr. Wangare told me that she had done some research on gender studies, focusing on issues of girl child education. It is not surprising therefore that she was one of those who seemed very keen to follow up on the issues we discussed in the interview.

Summary and Conclusion

This chapter has shown that Kenyan universities need to recognise the barriers within them that continue to hinder women's advancement. This has especially become urgent due to the emerging challenges presented by HIV and AIDS, which I discuss in the chapters that follow.

Women, too, need to be aware of institutional practices, cultures and ethos that hinder their career progression. An awareness of these issues can be achieved through research on women's issues. Through research findings, women may begin to reflect and talk about the hurdles they face, thus breaking the silence about their positions in the academy. Research can also act as a tool for theorising and strategising on workable approaches that would make universities women-friendly. The chapter has shown the need to find remedies to the unfairness caused by gender imbalance in the university context.

The discussions in this chapter suggest that, for women to manage a balance between their personal and professional roles, thus managing to compete on an equal footing with men, gender sensitive policies are required in Kenyan universities. The findings also indicate a need for universities to create spaces where women feel comfortable and thus able to perform to their best capabilities regardless of the demands on their personal selves (Wyn et al., 2000).

The issues raised by women in this study have shown that men can resist women entering 'their jobs.' This resistance is expressed in different ways that women may not discover easily. It can be by exclusion, and at other times through barriers that block women's advancement or through open harassment. There are even times when institutions change the rules to make it more difficult for women to succeed (see, for example, Dr. Wangare's experience in this chapter). Women are commonly "reminded of their 'natural' roles as wife, mother, and sexual partner" (Reskin, 2000: 264). Even those women who postpone marriage, run the 'risk' of failure to get husbands, and the constant reminder of ageing by their biological clock ticking (Reskin, 2000).

In order to make workplaces more accommodating to women, it would be useful for them to become active agents in challenging the status quo. One of the ways that women-friendly policies and programmes have been realised has been through an increased number of women (committed to feminism) in leadership positions (Wyn et al., 2000). In the following Chapter, I look at ways in which the absence of women's personal experiences in the public discourse may lead to their invisibility in policies and practices, especially those related to issues like HIV and AIDS.

= 7

Women's Experiences with HIV and AIDS: 'Back into the Personal'

Introduction

Stanley and Wise (1983), from whose article the second part of the title of this chapter is derived, note that they carry out research and write in a feminist way. A feminist way, according to them, is one that recognises the need to incorporate personal issues into the public domain.

The focus of this chapter is on the women's experiences with HIV and AIDS. The chapter attempts to answer the research question: How were senior women academic staff in Weruini and Holy Ghost universities affected by HIV and AIDS?

To answer this question, I asked women about their everyday experiences as affected by HIV and AIDS. These experiences, which lie in the 'personal', were the subject of this research. This was in appreciation of what Stanley and Wise (1983) note that what women spend their lives doing (even privately) "must be the subject of feminist research" (p. 195).

In Kenya, like other capitalist patriarchal societies, there is a separation of the public sphere from the private sphere (see Chapter Two). The two spheres are highly gendered, with the public spheres inhabited by men, who reap the benefits of socially valued activities such as politics and waged labour (Kiluva-Ndunda, 2001). Even when women occupy the public sphere (as was the case with the women in this study), they still perform much domestic labour (Deem, 2003; Tamale, 2005). This chapter suggests that the gendering and separation of the private and public sphere has contributed to the ways HIV and AIDS has affected the women interviewees.

Using data from conversational interviews with women, I show the need to take account of personal challenges when examining the university AIDS discourse. I explore the ways in which women's experiences can be used as a basis for gender sensitive AIDS policies and practices in the two universities studied. This chapter serves the purpose of breaking the silence around HIV and AIDS and its effects on senior women staff in the two universities. I also look at women's support systems when faced with challenges they talked about. Religion comes out as the main source of support, which I discuss in the final section of the chapter.

Women's Experiences as Affected by HIV and AIDS

I carried out this research on the premise that Kenyan universities have continued to be silent about the impact of HIV and AIDS on their staff members, especially senior staff (Kelly, 2001, 2003b; Nyutho et al., 2005; Nzioka, 2000). Indeed, women's personal experiences in universities seem unrecognised as studies have suggested (Currie et al., 2002; Grunberg, 2001; Lund, 1998; Morley and Walsh, 1996; Probert, 2005; Singh, 2003). The present study provided a platform where university women's experiences with HIV and AIDS were listened to and made public.

I am careful when I use the word 'listen'. hooks (1994) makes some observations that I find relevant to my objective of listening to women. In a dialogue, Ron Scapp, and bell hooks talk as follows:

Ron Scapp: Sometimes professors may even act as though personal recognition is important, but they do so in a superficial way. Professors, even those who view themselves as liberal, may think that it's good for students to speak, only to proceed in a manner that devalues what the students say.

Bell hooks: We are willing to hear Suzie speak even as we then immediately turn away from her words, erasing them… with that erasure Suzie is not able to see herself as a speaking subject worthy of voice…

Ron Scapp: In many classes, this comes full circle. In the end it is the teacher's voice that everyone knew all along was the only one to listen to… (hooks, 1994 p. 149-150).

Although this dialogue is about listening to students' voices in the classroom, I found their argument relevant to my research. I could have asked the women to talk about their experiences, but in coming to write, I turn away from them and not make them the central part of my discourse. I wanted the women to speak in my research and it is for this reason that I used some long extracts from the interviews. I have found it very difficult to edit what they said. I do not want to end up with my voice taking precedence over the women's voices. Their day-to-day experiences, away from the university, are brought back into the mainstream by becoming central to my writing. I am arguing that women's experiences with AIDS, in their homes and in the communities have an impact on them when they get to the universities.

Of the 20 women with whom I had conversational interviews, 15 had been affected by HIV and AIDS. Many of the women said that it was not easy to separate one's private life from office work, for example:

I think even if we want to separate our lives, that when we come to the office we can forget what is happening at home, it would be difficult. I may want to play an Ostrich game and forget about what happens at home, but I will not perform well. I remember when my sister-in-law was very sick and I came to work one morning and there was no concentration. I was to meet a colleague and I called and said: 'I am sorry today I cannot meet you because I have a patient at home'. So it has to affect you in one way or another. I don't think we can avoid it and even if it is not AIDS, there are other personal issues (Prof. Nyaboke, Weruini).

As the above statement indicates, it is difficult to separate the personal self from the public self. Prof. Nyaboke's point is that it is not possible for people to lead separate lives, one in the office and the other at home. The challenge is that not much research has been done to bring to light the private lives of Kenyan university women (see Chapter Six). There is a lot of research and writing on HIV and AIDS in Kenyan universities, but I have not come across any that focuses on how senior women in Kenyan universities are coping with the challenges of this pandemic either as affected or infected.

While the Kenyan workplaces treat the personal and the professional roles as separate entities, in a study of women and men managers in two Kenyan universities, Onsongo (2005) found that women managers found it difficult to separate private issues from office work and writes about an observation she made during her interview with one of the women managers. The woman received a telephone call from her husband informing her that their house help was ill and she needed to be taken to hospital. This woman was expected to take time off to sort out that domestic matter, but there was no such expectation on her husband.

Although the Kenyan workplaces are organised in ways where gender roles do not interfere with professional performance, this is not always easy as noted by Onsongo (2005) and Deem (2003) referring to UK universities. Even though several women in my study felt that they could not separate their private and public lives, there lacked spaces in the universities where the private issues could be expressed, as is indicated from the following statement from one of my respondents:

I am very social and I would like to be with people, but here I noticed you have to go slow, you have to weigh whom you will talk to because you find people are business-minded. I do not like the attitude. I have learnt to adapt to it although I would wish things were different where one felt there was some support at work. After all, this is the place where we spend most of our time. I know this lack of concern for people's lives is a problem because apart from HIV and AIDS, there are other social issues... I don't like this kind of atmosphere where people behave as though they have no personal problems and yet we all have problems (Mrs Bihanya , Lecturer, Weruini).

Many women in my study said that they would appreciate if the universities could recognise their personal problems, even though not directly related to their work. Going by what many women in this study were saying, it would be useful if workplaces created spaces for staff members to talk and deal with their private selves. The data in this study suggests that women affected by HIV and AIDS may find such spaces useful, as noted by Mrs Bihanya and in similar studies by others (Leonard, 2001; Mabokela, 2003; Morley, 1999).

HIV and AIDS are associated with painful feelings and expressing them is not always easy (Rankka, 1998). I am arguing that if universities do not provide space where these experiences are expressed, this could lead to "destruction of self-purpose, individual or collective brokenness, self hatred, loss of agency and hope and could culminate in despair" (p. 51). The muting of women's experiences in African universities is what Barnes (2005: 9) likens to lack of 'air time' for women in academia.

According to Barnes (2005), male academics "are centre stage, in the spotlight, with the microphone" (p. 9). My study was conducted with the aim of giving women 'the microphone' to voice their experiences with HIV and AIDS. Following are some other voices from affected women in the academia:

I lost my two brothers and it is a trauma because I remember the first death... of course we knew once you are HIV positive you are dying. So the trauma of imagining this person is going to die and there is nothing you can do about it was too much. There was that initial trauma and running up and down taking them to hospital, trying to get them to eat the right foods. Then finally they died. The permanence of death just hurts. I must say the experience has been painful but I would say mine has been even more painful because my two brothers died in consecutive years. And these were young people (Dr. Atoti, Senior Lecturer, Weruini).

I was most affected by my kid brother. First of all because he's a kid brother, I mean this is a baby and you can't help but wonder 'where did I fail or abandon him to make this happen to him?' When he's sitting there he's hungry and you give him food and he cannot swallow. That is painful. The last time I saw him he was lying on the couch and I walked in, he wanted to tell me something but he couldn't talk then he said: 'It's okay' that was on a Saturday afternoon and he passed on the following day in the afternoon. What hit me most was the fact that I couldn't do anything for him, which is not nice. It isn't nice at all because you want to help the ones you love when they are incapacitated. It just killed me to imagine what he went through and the fact that I could not help him (Prof Atieno, Weruini).

Some of the expressions in the above statements show anger and the pain that these women went through as they watched their loved ones die of AIDS. Their families and communities view these women as those who should provide support. Expectations that women should provide care and support for family members during times of need, ranging from child care, care for the sick, and for the elderly, to students, are not unique to Kenya as studies in other parts of the world suggest (Beechey and Whitelegg, 1986; Coleman, 2002; Hatt, 1999b; Hughes, et al., 2005; Mavin and Bryans, 2002; McKie et al., 2001; McKie et al., 2004; Miroiu, 2003; Onsongo, 2000). Two other women said:

Yes I am affected. My sister realised her husband had HIV and he didn't tell her. He told the doctor to tell her. She wanted to commit suicide because they had been having unprotected sex... the man knew he had HIV and he never told her. He said that because she delivered through caesarean, she is the one who brought HIV. I took her for a test ...she didn't want anybody to know. So I used my name when she gave her blood... she was tested and she was negative but the man has since passed away. When I learnt of it the first time, I just broke down and cried (Mrs Wandera, Lecturer, Holy Ghost University).

My elder sister is HIV positive... It took the family quite some time before we realised she was positive. ... She is really struggling. Every time she's down and up. It is really working on all of us. It impacted on us very badly because this was a lady we looked up to as a role model... It really dealt a blow to all of us. Our self-esteem was really affected... you know the way some of these self-esteems are arranged on one another. Even as an individual, it messed up my self-esteem and I have really struggled to accept my family. I still feel angry and it pains me a lot (Mrs Kibet, Counsellor, HG University).

Mrs Wandera talked about shielding her sister by 'pretending' that she (Mrs Wandera) was the one being tested for HIV and not her sister. This shows the extent of the stigma associated with HIV and AIDS and the lengths people can go to conceal their identity (see also Chapter Nine). In Mrs Kibet's case, her sister's problems affected the self-esteem of the whole family. Mrs Kibet would be hesitant about letting others know of her sister's problems, especially working at Holy Ghost University where the expectation is for them to live up to Christian values (see Chapter Eight).

This feeling of shame is not restricted to HIV and AIDS alone. Wickham-Searl (1992) notes that stigma of children's disability can be transferred to caring mothers. Mrs Kibet was referring to the shame and stigma she felt for her family to have a sister suffering from AIDS. The discourse of silence in the wider community also leads to silence in the university as the staff feel ashamed to reveal that they are affected by AIDS (see more on silence and shame in Chapter Nine).

There were no differences between the experiences of the women from Holy Ghost and those from Weruini. They had all experienced AIDS in their families and the pain was similar. I was particularly concerned about Holy Ghost where the dean, who also happened to be the head of the AIDS Control Unit, said that their staff had nothing to do with AIDS because they adhered to Christian values. The dean appeared to be unaware of the pain that some of the women were going through. Yet some people in Holy Ghost University may have been infected, a fact noted by their deputy human resource manager (see Chapter Eight) while all the women I interviewed were affected.

In Weruini, there was acknowledgment that the problem of AIDS existed. However, there was no mention from the administration of ways in which staff members were dealing with the pain and loss and how these may have affected their work. The attitude was that staff members were somehow coping with the effects of the epidemic, or even, were untouched by its effects.

The lack of awareness of women's private experiences in both Weruini and Holy Ghost could be linked to the predominant patriarchal culture in the universities. On this I find McKie et al.'s (2004) assertion appropriate, that:

> …feminist theoretical analyses have sought to critique, first, the artificial separation of instrumental and expressive tasks, which ignores the organisational and managerial components of domestic work, second, the division between the public and the private that forms the basis of many policies and services. Such a division denies the blurring of boundaries between the public world of paid employment and the private sphere of domestic life that allows the aspects of the public to intrude into the home and expects the private to prop up and cement the vulnerabilities of the public (p. 596).

The two universities in my study were lacking opportunities where senior staff members could talk about their personal issues. McKie at al. (2004) further note that many institutions fail to consider the interrelated nature of public and private spheres. Nonetheless, public vision is influenced by domestic vision and indeed private behaviour is also influenced by public actions like family policies. Other researchers, for example Brannen et al. (1994), Coleman (2002) and Probert (2005) imply that whenever the private and the public arenas behave as though they are unrelated, the people who get mostly affected are women.

However, writers like Wisker (1996) hold a different view; that it may be useful to separate work from other personal activities in order to have something different to hold on to "should disaster strike" (p. 140). Wisker (1996) argues that some balance can be achieved by maintaining a home life, which provides an escape from work demands, or work life, which provides an escape from home. Nonetheless the findings of my study suggest that, for women, home may not always be an escape from work. Thus, home and professional work could not be separated. This leads me to the next section where I look at the actual responsibilities that the women in my study said they had taken when AIDS struck in their families.

Gender, Care and AIDS

Fifteen women in my sample who said that they were directly affected by HIV and AIDS (meaning immediate family members had been infected), had cared for or were still caring for someone who was infected. The other five who said they were not directly affected were also involved in providing some kind of care either to their communities, their church members or to their extended families. All the women I interviewed, therefore, had cared for or were still caring for people who were infected or affected by HIV and AIDS.

For many years, the international debate about caring for people with AIDS has focused on what is commonly referred to as 'home-based care' (GHC, 2005; Kelly, 2003; Lipinge et al., 2004). This care is obviously seen to be viable in countries ravaged by the epidemic because it is less expensive in situations where hospitals can no longer cope with the large numbers of people who may have no hope of recovering.

Home-based care is useful when resources are scarce. But it has meant that women bear the burden of looking after the sick (UNAIDS, 2004b). The burden placed on women is hardly recognised in workplace policies and practices. On the issue of home-based care, Barnett and Whiteside (2002) note:

> ... our extended family will cope with orphans', people used to say in Africa in the 1990's ... it is necessary to find ways to care for orphans within the family and the household systems that have been increasingly stretched, using institutional care as a last resort (p. 207).

Barnett and Whiteside (2002) further note that what seems to be ignored is that it is actually women and girls who provide this home-based care. Many societies have not considered compensating these women, or having workplace policies that take this care work into consideration, yet the alternative would be to place ailing people into institutional care, which is expensive. This whole debate, that the extended family will cope, is another way that governments transfer key societal responsibilities to women (and girls). This point was expounded by the women, as shown in one of the interview abstracts below:

> I have been affected so much by HIV ... For example, when I was working in another university before I came here, I used to live in a friend's house. Her husband had AIDS. On his last days he was very ill. He got cancer and my friend and I had to look after him 24 hours, as he was bedridden. It was hard for us. He eventually died after suffering in terrible pain for a few months. We were both devastated. My sister's husband was also sick at the same time. He had been sick for a long time. I had helped her to take care of him because they lived here in Nairobi... I did not realise he was dying of AIDS until my sister told me. She also started to waste away. By the time we were burying her husband after Easter holidays of 1998, she was also wasting very

fast and we buried her in August, the same year. Then later on, my brother got sick... there were financial constraints and every time we had to raise money to pay the hospital bills...I suffered emotionally. I could not concentrate with my work. I was all over – in class teaching, analysing the PhD data half way, going to hospital or communicating to my brothers who are out of Nairobi and telling them the progress. I was also seeing my father who was devastated after my sister passed away. It made me lose a whole year and a half on my PhD. I did very little so I just left my data collection at that point. I picked up again last year (Mrs Bihanya, Lecturer, Weruini).

A closer look at what Mrs Bihanya is saying shows a gender dimension in care provision, both emotional and physical. Mrs Bihanya told me that she has a number of older brothers. But she was the one who had to care and support her sister and the brother in law until they both died. She was the overall coordinator of activities involving the sick siblings. In addition, she had to provide emotional support for her parents who were deeply affected after the death of their daughter. All these responsibilities led her to halt her PhD studies for a year and a half.

Research which has looked at the gender dimensions of providing care in the family, for example, Finch and Mason (1993) has shown that both men and women suggested that women were particularly good at certain kinds of family responsibilities. In the Finch and Mason's study there were twice as many examples of women providing personal care than men. Besides HIV and AIDS, which was the focus of this study, other caring responsibilities were also mentioned, for example:

You know my mother-in-law got sick. She got a stroke. She never used to walk and she had to be carried around because she used to live with me in my house. She was worse than a baby. That was about four years ago and I was also sick. I needed an operation and I pleaded with somebody to look after her and they refused. In fact, we told the doctor to keep her in hospital because I had come from hospital myself. I looked after her for three years. Can you imagine? The first girl I

employed to look after her left after one week. Later I got others who
assisted me. But it was still a big challenge and I couldn't concentrate
much on my work. She eventually died. Her sickness really affected
my work (Mrs Wakaba, Lecturer Weruini).

Mrs Wakaba talked of how she shelved her plans to write a PhD
proposal due to her own illness and that of her mother-in-law. This
is another example of gender-specific care work. Mrs Wakaba, for
example, did not mention the part played by her husband even
though it was his mother requiring care. In Chapter Six, I argue
that research on women's issues is one way of creating awareness
on issues that women and men take for granted. These caring
responsibilities were extended beyond immediate family members
as noted by a woman academic in the following statement:

> I am not affected directly because HIV has not infected any member of
> my nuclear family – or rather there is none that I know about. But in
> the extended family, we have lost quite a number of married couples
> that have left children behind. I think I am affected like everybody
> else because I am taking care of three orphans. One is about nine and
> when the mother died she said I should be the one to look after her
> because I seemed to care when she was sick. Although she did not
> know she was going to die, she had indicated that in case she dies, I
> should take care of the daughter. So I took the daughter six years ago
> and I've been taking care of her. She doesn't live with me here but she
> lives with my mother. It was difficult for me to transfer her because
> she had identified with my mother. Then I have two other girls who
> are related to my husband. The parents also died and we were given
> the responsibility to look after them. In the extended family of aunties
> and the uncles, I think there are over 20 orphans who we have to help
> (Mrs. Kibaata, Chaplain, HG).

Mrs Kibaata talked about the double requirement created by
her job as a pastor since people expected her to support them even
when they were not related to her. In her church work, she comes
across numerous people infected with HIV and AIDS, many of

them in their dying stages. She has received requests from such women to look after their children after their death. At the time of the interview, Mrs Kibaata was supporting a group of orphans living in a slum where her church is located. She said for many years it was difficult to talk about AIDS in the church (the issue of church support and lack of it in some cases is addressed in Chapter Seven), but she had support from NGOs.

The expectation that women will combine full-time employment with other social responsibilities seems to cut across many cultures as noted by Hughes et al. (2005):

> Caring work is seen as the responsibility of women and to take part in such work is linked 'umbilically' to their social and economic role. Care policy is premised on the notion that such work will be the responsibility of women... there is evidence to suggest that the gendered nature of caring work, both paid and unpaid, reinforces already existing inequalities in the labour market (p. 261).

As the above quotation indicates, the gender inequalities in the labour market can be explained by the time spent by women on domestic responsibilities. Probert (2005) observes that besides unequal treatment between men and women in universities, women also have to contend with greater responsibilities for family work, which may have an impact on their careers.

Caring, love and affection are seen to be important factors in determining how people, especially women, define their self-identities. However, work undertaken within the home and family continues to be seen as non-work (McKie et al., 2001). This is not just because it is not paid for, but also because it is seen to be borne out of love and affection and contained within duty and obligation (Delphy and Leonard, 1992; Leonard and Speakman, 1986; McKie et al., 2004).

Ambivalence exists amongst policy makers, employers, and society more generally, towards the gendered nature of caring and the implications of this for employed women (McKie et al., 2001). Universities continue to operate within patriarchal systems and structures that leave no space for private discourses, yet women's lack of progression is normally blamed on the lack of individual initiative, ambition and on laziness (Kamau, 2002; Onsongo, 2000).

Literature on the gender dimensions of care work and their effect on the labour market, indicate that caring work requires complex negotiations around assumptions about gender roles and responsibilities both within and outside the home (Boyd, 2002; Finch and Mason, 1993; Fogelberg et al., 1999; Humpreys and Gutenby, 1999; Kjeldal, 2005; McKie et al., 2001; McKie et al., 2004; Probert, 2005; Warren, 2003; Wickham-Searl, 1992). These negotiations would be useful in coming up with some support systems that people can resort to when faced with personal challenges that affect their careers.

In the following section, I discuss the role of religion as a support for women. In Chapter Eight I compare the considerable support accorded to university students, especially by women staff, while the women receive no support.

"Support from God"

The findings discussed in this chapter suggest that women respondents were faced with challenges that may not have been experienced by their male colleagues (see also Deem, 2003). To survive, they too required some support. I was interested to find out where women sought support for themselves having provided support to others.

When I asked the women in my study where they derive their support from, all except one said, "I get my strength and support from God". In this section, I analyse the issue of religion as a source of support for women during times of difficulty.

Supporting those with AIDS has been seen by both the providers of support and those receiving it as a "response of love which is real and life-giving as AIDS is real and death bringing" (Kelly,

2003: 8-9). As I have argued so far, women form the majority of those providing this support. Caring for terminally ill patients can be extremely draining to the carer as Kelly (2003) notes:

> Caregivers are in regular contact with death and the death of relatively young people. This situation can drain human energy and generate sadness, even anger. We must admit that we all are wounded and burdened. We have a duty to ourselves, our families and our patients, to make sure of some rest time, of proper food, of a chance to share our burdens and problems with a compassionate listener (p. 8-9).

While the women in my study were not in full-time care work, as those Kelly is addressing in the above quotation, they too require support to handle the difficult challenges that come with caring and living with AIDS patients (as pointed out earlier in this chapter). The problem for educated women is that they are not likely to be viewed by the Kenyan society as requiring support. They are financially able and are thought to be in control of their lives. This could lead to a denial of their needs for support.

I was interested in finding out whether their universities were seen as a source of support during difficult times in their private domain. None of the women said they received any direct support from their university. This was partly because they did not officially communicate with the universities about these difficulties. However, none of them was aware of any available channels in the university that they could use to address personal issues (see Chapter Eight).

In Kenya, the role of religion when people are faced with matters of life and death cannot be underestimated, as I pointed out in Chapter Two. Spiritual involvement plays an important role in lives of terminally ill people and those caring for them (Ciambrone, 2003). However, I did not expect that senior university women would be that deeply committed to religion and that it was their main source of support.

It has been documented that, in general terms, it is people who are socially weak or legally powerless who tend to find more solace from religion (Elkins, 2005; Shelp and Sunderland, 1987). In the United States, for example, it has been observed that religious involvement seems to be especially important for black and Latina women (Sosnowitz 1995 quoted in Ciambrone, 2003). Religion does seem to help those already disadvantaged in other ways to cope with life stresses.

In Chapter Two, I discussed ways in which the patriarchal structures have kept Kenyan women in positions that make them legally and socially powerless and disadvantaged. Even though women may feel comfortable seeking solace in religion, I argue that institutional support structures that could be of assistance where the church may not help would be useful in the two universities. It is also important to acknowledge that there are people who are not affiliated to any religious institutions.

None of the women mentioned that universities provided any support. The only support that could remotely be linked to the universities was that of colleagues, which was mainly informal rather than institutional (see Chapter Eight).

Interviews with the women suggest that the same church that supports them may let them down, when a problem like AIDS strikes. A mixture of compassion and condemnation of the infected has influenced the modern Kenyan churches' response to diseases like AIDS (Gichure, 2006). This attitude of condemnation from the same church that offers support was shared by two of the women in my study as shown in the following extracts:

> Most of my strength came from my inner self and from God. Often I would break down and cry and when I came out of it, I could talk to people. When my brother was very sick and unable to walk, he sometimes asked me to ask the priest to come and pray for him in the house. He was unable to walk to the church, which is only five minutes away from my house (we are staunch Catholics). But after sharing with the priest about his problem, I realised he was not really concerned – his concern was really superficial. I realised it was only us relatives who could fully understand the pain our brother was going

through. I don't know whether it was the weakness of this particular priest, but my church did not offer as much support as I expected (Mrs Bihanya, Lecturer, Weruini).

Of course, the Church has also been quite supportive, but HIV/AIDS apparently is one of the areas where Church members would not want to get directly involved. In the past, I was alone in AIDS work. My colleagues used to wonder 'how can a whole Church Minister with a master's degree work with those people'. They would ask 'Have you missed something better to do? Why do kazi ya uchafu, kazi ya prostitutes' (she was seen to be doing dirty work, working with prostitutes) (Mrs Kibaata, Chaplain, HG).

The above two women presented the paradox of the church's response to this pandemic. Despite the fact that the church has been known to be intolerant towards people with AIDS, an issue that I return to in the following chapter, it has also played a key role in peer support and counselling for the infected (Ciambrone, 2003). Among the women in Ciambrone's sample, spirituality appeared to be an important coping strategy. Likewise, several women in my study found solace in the Church. HIV and AIDS present people with pain that can only be healed in a place that they find safe (Ciambrone, 2003). The discussions I had with the women suggest that in order for people to freely share their experiences on HIV and AIDS, they require an atmosphere of openness and acceptance. According to a majority of the women in my study, such an environment was found within their Christian communities and fellowships:

My biggest support comes first and foremost from God because you must get some courage and insight to be able to deal with such things. In our Church, we have programmes related to HIV and AIDS so, at least, I have those I can run to and tell them this is what is happening, how do I get help? (Ms. Karabo, Lecturer, HG).

I am a Christian and I have a heavy reliance on God and even the days I don't feel Him very close to me, I know He's there. I can go and rave and make noise the whole day and His word will still be there and at that time of my brother's illness and death, I comforted myself with the Lord's words that 'my place is sufficient for you'. Some people may think this is defeatist, but I disagree. ...so the support I got from the word of God was great (Prof Atieno, Weruini).

At my own personal level, I derive my support mostly from God. I am a born again Christian so all my strength comes from my relationship with God (Mrs Musoga, Lecturer, Weruini).

Yes, you know when you are a human being you are nothing without God. When challenges come, you cannot handle them alone. You hand them over to God. So it is like a partnership with God, everything. Like I told you, I am a counsellor, although I have not been trained as one but there are some things I do better than the experts because of my partnership with God... (Mrs Wakaba, Lecturer, HG).

All the women in my study (except Dr. Wangare) used the word God at some point in the interview. Sentiments like those shown in the extracts above were common right across the board. Even where there were disappointments with the church, the women still felt that turning to God and to prayer offered them support that they could not get elsewhere.

In her study of women and men managers in two Kenyan universities, Onsongo (2005) also notes how her research participants pointed to the importance of their Christian faith in overcoming challenges they faced as managers. In the context of HIV and AIDS, the reliance on God can be interpreted to show the sense of helplessness facing many of those affected by the epidemic.

Strong ties to religion may lead to problems of stigma and silence that I discuss in Chapter Nine. The church's handling of certain issues like homosexuality and gender can also pose some barriers in AIDS work and prevention (see Chapter Nine). I argue that alternative support systems need to be created and institutionalised for effective management of a problem like HIV and AIDS. This can be done without dismissing religion as important way of helping people to cope (Ciambrone, 2003).

Summary and Conclusion

The discussions in this chapter suggest that HIV and AIDS epidemic can be used to expose and explore silences and indifferences about gender inequalities that have existed in universities for many years. Using feminist concepts of care and the 'personal as political', I have analysed women's experiences with HIV and AIDS. Their stories suggest the need to develop an AIDS' discourse in universities, which recognises that professional women's lives are affected and influenced by their private lives.

It is possible that when women spend much of their time in activities that are not career enhancing, they may suffer long-term disadvantages. It would help if these activities were acknowledged in mainstream university practices. The women's experiences showed that in the two universities studied, there was no acknowledgement of the challenges senior women staff faced in relation to HIV and AIDS.

This chapter has shown that a lack of dialogue between the private and the public, mainly affects women who bear the burden of private responsibilities. This lack of support for women was found to create hurdles to women's career progression as shown in Chapter Six and in this chapter. Support for women was found to be mainly spiritual as many of them said they relied on God and prayer to cope. Spirituality is an emotion-focused strategy and it clearly helps people to cope psychologically (Ciambrone, 2003). However, there is need for other more effective and practical ways of helping people cope.

The present chapter suggests that a discourse of HIV and AIDS awareness in universities need not be 'one-dimensional', focusing only on the dramatic spread and devastating impact of HIV and

AIDS on those who are infected or viewed as being at risk of infection. Rather, an AIDS discourse requires a deeper analysis of the inter-related factors. These include gender issues, patriarchy and a recognition that social challenges like AIDS, which fall in the private domain, need to be recognised and acted on in the public discourses which inform policies. I address these issues further in the following chapter.

= 8

'Maybe Next Year': Impact and Responses to HIV and AIDS in the Sample Universities

I really do not know if anything is happening here. I tend to think that there is quite a bit of silence because I don't think there is a forum where such things are addressed. Secondly, I know there are people who have died of AIDS-related causes but we just feel sorry and mourn just like we would mourn any other death. Honestly, I am not aware of any programme here dealing with issues of HIV and AIDS specifically targeting staff members

– Mrs Bahati, Lecturer, Holy Ghost University

Introduction

I derived the phrase, 'maybe next year' from a chapter by Treichler and Warren (1998). They note that feminists were silent about the impact of HIV and AIDS on women during the early years of the pandemic. The attitude held by feminists towards AIDS, as noted by Treichler and Warren (1998) is similar to what this study found in the two universities. There is evidence that HIV and AIDS has had considerable impact on Kenyan universities (CHE and UNESCO, 2004). This impact has been in terms of loss of staff and students, reduced productivity, direct and indirect costs, strain on facilities and on quality of service (Owino, 2004).

At the time of this study, it was noted that Kenyan universities are at different levels of putting up responses to this scourge, but many of them still lacked systematic impact and risk assessment (Kelly, 2004b). In this chapter, I address the research question: How had the two universities responded to the impact of HIV and AIDS on their senior women staff? I start the chapter by discussing AIDS impact in Weruini and Holy Ghost as seen by the women and the management. I then provide an analysis of the responses taken by the two universities, with a focus on Weruini AIDS policy. In the final part of the chapter I compare the support (HIV and AIDS related and other non-academic) given to students in the two universities with the apparent lack of support for senior women staff.

Impact of HIV and AIDS in the two Universities

The impact of epidemics usually creates history-changing events (Barnett and Whiteside, 2002). This is because some lives are terminated and others are incapacitated as the affected people divert energy and time into care. AIDS increases sickness and deaths in populations at young ages where normal levels of sickness and death are low. Due to high rates of sickness and death, other impacts follow.

In the case of universities, the impacts that follow include; loss of staff and students, reduced productivity, strain on facilities, reduced morale, and strain on quality (Kelly, 2001; 2004b). In addition, as the findings of this study suggest, the impact may also increase gender inequalities in universities. This is because women make up the majority of those who divert their energy and time into care in addition to being more vulnerable to HIV infection (Roth and Hogan, 1998; Waller, 2004; Wood, 2002).

I wanted to establish the AIDS impact on the universities for two reasons. First, I believe that in order to have appropriate responses, the impact needs to be understood. Secondly, ignoring the impact of an epidemic like AIDS would be counterproductive to the universities' development goals and prospects for progress, especially related to gender equality. From the interviews with women and management, I got the impression that there was not much appreciation of AIDS impact on senior staff in the two universities. The women talked about their experiences at personal level, but they were not sure of what was happening to their colleagues. Ignorance or general lack of concern on the side of the management about the impact of this epidemic on senior staff could be linked to the high level of secrecy, denial and fear of discrimination about HIV and AIDS apparent in the two universities (see also Chapter Nine).

During the focused interviews, I talked to those people who were either involved in HIV and AIDS work or holding positions that could make them aware of the impact this epidemic had on their institutions. Of the five managers that I interviewed, two were the directors of the AIDS Control Units (ACU) in the two universities. The rest comprised a deputy human resources manager at Holy Ghost, a member of the board of directors (ACU, Weruini), and the Vice Chancellor of Weruini.

To my surprise, even people working directly with HIV and AIDS displayed little concern about the social challenges that their staff faced. The only awareness seemed to revolve around medical aspects of the epidemic. The male managers talked about sickness, absenteeism and deaths among their staff. Although interviews with the women revealed experiences of emotional stress and caring responsibilities, those in management (except the only woman manager as I show later in this chapter) seemed unaware of the inside stories narrated by the women.

In the following sub-sections, I look at how the management of Weruini and Holy Ghost viewed the impact of HIV and AIDS in their universities. I also analyse the difference that was clear in the perception of the only woman manager compared to the four men.

Impact in Weruini

As I listened to what women and management said was the impact, I found that the university discourse was dominated by patriarchy (see Chapter Two for a definition of patriarchy). The Kenyan society organises its affairs to cater for and sustain male supremacy over women. I have also noted that patriarchy in Kenya has its roots in long established traditions of male dominance, which have made the male perspective the social perspective. Male managers in Weruini and Holy Ghost viewed AIDS from a male perspective. Both universities had male directors for their AIDS Control Units. None of the women I interviewed said they were involved in AIDS work in their universities.

The following are some extracts of what the managers saw as the impact of HIV and AIDS in Weruini University:

> We have had several deaths of staff members, particularly the subordinate staff. We suspect they die of AIDS-related complications but we are never sure. When it comes to senior members of staff, we sometimes lose one a year or so…it becomes difficult to know whether they have died of AIDS-related illnesses…There is absenteeism of those who have lost loved ones; staff who are ailing and so on. So that has affected performance. It's not unusual for a member of staff to seek permission to be away for a whole week, without any clarification of why they need to be away…Another thing, of course, is that when these people are bed-ridden, they cannot be dismissed from the university because they are sick. When they are away, they still occupy their positions (Dr. Oduor, ACU Director, Weruini).

> As you know, universities are intricately structured and within that structure we have the main activities some of which are taken care of by particular departments… from the 1990s particularly starting in 1995 to date, there has been a rise in the number of AIDS victims, students and staff, so the university became more concerned about the threat of AIDS. Another thing that we noticed is the low productivity of staff when that malaise hits them, they go down and, therefore, absences are evident. … In fact, it's something that's throughout Africa whereby it attacks the most productive people. So the university's productivity was definitely undermined by that … the university has suffered great losses since medical bills keep going up… (Prof Atwoli, Weruini).

Both men in the above cited statements mention that there are deaths, which may be difficult to associate with AIDS. Absenteeism was also another impact in Weruini.

One of the challenges that AIDS has presented to workplaces in Africa is non-attendance (Barnett and Whiteside, 2002; Phaswana-Mafuya and Peltzer, 2006). Absenteeism may not only result from illness, but it also affects those attending funerals or those tending ailing family members. The other problem that AIDS has presented is unproductive staff. Barnett and Whiteside (2002) note that sick "employees may force themselves to work because if they don't they will lose their jobs" (p. 245). However, absenteeism due to sickness is said to have reduced in places where AIDS treatment has been scaled up (Lindow, 2006; UNAIDS, 2005). I discuss the situation of AIDS treatment in Weruini later on in this chapter.

Prof Atwoli also refers to those infected as 'victims', a term seen to reflect a negative attitude (Gichure, 2006). Persons with AIDS were initially called AIDS victims. This was a medical term that viewed AIDS as a plague and those who got it were victims. Victimisation of people only aggravated the stigmatisation. However, as more people contracted AIDS and the more doctors and social workers listened to their stories, the less they were seen as victims (Gichure, 2006). In addition, Gichure (2002) observes that:

A victim is one who is afflicted unjustly. A victim is powerless/ voiceless and always at the mercy of the oppressor. This is not what AIDS is. AIDS has no cure but it does not make us worthless. It should not make us shameful nor should it be an occasion for passing judgement on people's integrity. People with AIDS are still valuable and have a contribution to make to the society. Today it is generally accepted that people with AIDS should be referred to as 'people living with AIDS' (p. 120).

The use of the word 'victim' could therefore be interpreted to mean that the attitude among Weruini management leans towards stigmatisation, an issue that I explore further in Chapter Nine.

Although Weruini management was aware of a serious threat of AIDS to the institution, especially due to absenteeism from work, there was no mention of the impact of the pandemic on the individual lives of staff members. There seemed to be no plans to involve people at a more personal level in order to understand how this disease was affecting them as individuals. I listened with interest when Prof. Atwoli was explaining how universities were 'intricately structured' and how things were done according to these structures.

Prof Atwoli gave me an impression of someone with a structured outlook and he believed in following the laid down procedures. Throughout the interview, he had the university AIDS policy, and he kept looking at it, in a way making sure that what he said did not contradict the policy. He is the only interviewee who requested for the interview schedule beforehand so that he could prepare himself. He seemed keen to be 'politically correct'. None of the women requested to be given the interview schedule in advance. I gave him the schedule as requested aware of the fact that this could introduce bias, but since the questions were very general in nature, I did not see much risk in having him look at the questions in advance.

Women's voices can easily disappear within these university structures and environment, which Leonard (2001) describes as having:

> An academic professionality...embedded with them an antagonism, a project of masculinity, of (super) rationality, of scientism, of independence which attempts to keep safe and secure and strong by keeping or driving out or denying elements associated with femininity (emotions, bodies,...personal interconnections) (p. 43).

Elements associated with femininity, which the women interviewees talked about (see Chapter Seven), may have no place in these professional [patriarchal] structures. This was implied by Dr. Oduor (quoted above), whose concern was about the loss of working time due to the days taken by those attending funerals. The two men (Oduor and Atwoli) seemed unaware of the challenges that women in their university could have been facing owing to the responsibilities that they take when family members fall ill. Women may not just be absent to attend funerals, but are also more involved long before the funerals because they take care of HIV and AIDS patients.

There was no mention of the impact on people's feelings and emotions, which were central amongst all the women interviewed. The position taken by the two men representing Weruini management can be linked to what Oakley (2001) refers to when she argues that universities are becoming like "factories with tightly timetabled and controlled culture, supervised by managers and bosses whose prime concern is with discrete and easily quantifiable deliverables..." (p. xi). In these university structures, women's needs may easily become obscured by what is generally seen as a gender-neutral environment.

In her literature search about the mechanisms that operate in African universities which have perpetuated personal and professional identities and institutional practices of gender inequality, Barnes (2005) argues that this inequality results from the fact that African men were admitted to universities much earlier than women. This created a gender gap that has persisted to the time I was carrying out this study.

Barnes (2005) further notes that African universities have also operated with gendered post-colonial dynamics that have led issues that affect women to be excluded from the mainstream. Male dominance in African universities, according to Barnes (2005) "has also created a resistance, if not hostility, to changing the norms of the 'club' to accommodate the perspectives and needs of women as students and staff" (p. 5). Male dominance was apparent in both Weruini and Holy Ghost, contributing to 'invisibility' of women's needs and perspectives.

In Chapter One I noted that educated women's voices as either affected or infected are absent in the AIDS discourse. This absence of women's issues is not unique to African universities as noted by Davies (1996) when she traces the concept of professionalism and bureaucracy in the West:

> Women's struggles to enter the professions in the late 19th century and early 20th century...were not just a matter of doors and minds being closed to women, but of the values that were embedded in the notion of the practices of a profession reflecting a masculine project and repressing or denying those qualities culturally assigned to femininity (p. 669).

The 'opening' of professional doors referred to by Davies (1996) seems to be echoed in the Kenyan context, where workplace norms have little room for values and qualities that are important to women (see Chapter 2). Universities reflect the cultures of the context in which they operate (Bond, 2000). In the era of AIDS, this has meant that the experiences discussed in Chapter 7 may have no place in a professional setting where people are expected to perform and produce results without bringing in their personal problems.

According to Barnes (2005), African universities have failed to accept and work with the prevailing facts. This is the fact of the multiple burdens that face women students and staff, and who need to deal with both their professional/learning lives and the logistics of their family lives.

Impact in Holy Ghost

AIDS impact in this Christian university was viewed in a slightly different way from Weruini. This is in line with Bond's (2000) argument that:

> ... the deeply embedded assumptions and values inherent in an institution are derived from its institutional history, size, age, and reputation and whether it is public or private, religious or secular... (p. 80).

A similar point is noted by Deem (2003), when she observes that the type of institution influenced the career narratives given by male and female managers in her study. In her case, the differences in the institutions were the 'post and pre-1992' universities in the UK. In my study, the differences in the two institutions were private/ religious and public/secular (see Chapter Three).

It seems that the Christian values guiding Holy Ghost University influence the official position taken regarding HIV and AIDS:

> I cannot say there has been a big impact, at least not among our staff. But because our students come from the same schools as those who go to public universities where the epidemic has been viewed as taking

a toll on quite a big chunk of the population, then we have to be concerned about HIV/AIDS awareness. We must be able to offer some help and some advice to the students but not staff whom we recruit with care and we expect them to maintain high moral standards... (Dr. Kivuu, ACU Director, HG).

Dr. Kivuu's position was that there was no HIV and AIDS amongst staff because they all adhere to Christian values (see Chapter Four). According to him, HIV was only a concern because of their students who come from the "same schools as those in public universities" where they may have contracted the disease. This is why the university has taken an interest in creating awareness amongst the students, but, apparently, there was no problem with staff. Focus on students and leaving out staff in South African universities has also been noted by Phaswana-Mafuya (2006).

Dr. Kivuu's account was contradicted by the deputy human resource manager, a woman, who said that the situation was different because she knew that some of their staff may have been HIV positive. Mrs Mwala saw the human faces behind this pandemic, not just the numbers of those who miss work. Her position at the human resources department made it easier for her to know about the personal issues of staff; for example, leave requests, medical problems, and loan applications:

> To talk about AIDS is not easy because as you know there is stigma. Most of the time you will not even know who has it or who has died of it. It is not very easy because there is no one who will come out and say he has it but somehow, I know because I am dealing with the medical scheme. There are very few cases...I could guess those who go for medical check-ups because we get the reports. They are not many. Very few ...they used to be many but you know we have gone through restructuring. Maybe they could be around ten this is my guess (Mrs Mwala, deputy human resource manager, HG).

Mrs Mwala's response here touches on silence and stigma, which I discuss in Chapter Nine. I use this extract here to show that a woman manager was aware of the reality that people in Holy

Ghost were affected just like anyone else. She said that the numbers of those infected in Holy Ghost might have reduced because there was staff retrenchment a year before my study. There had been suspicions that some of those retrenched may have been known to be HIV positive (see also further below in this chapter). Mrs Mwala knew that the attitude of management was that a disease associated with sinners should not affect Christians.

At the beginning of the interview, Mrs Mwala was more silent. This changed as our conversation progressed after I also spoke to her about my own experiences with HIV and AIDS and the silence I had witnessed at my university (also a Christian one). She became relaxed and began to speak more openly. For example, I had asked her if she knew of any staff members who may have been affected, she responded to this question towards the end of the interview by commenting:

> ... ooh you had asked if there are people who are also affected. Yes there are and even some staff members' spouses have died. There are two ladies whose husbands had passed away earlier so we are trying to see how their children can be helped. We are trying to gather the final dues and use them well so that they can be helped... Last year we had a staff member whose spouse had that problem and you know their productivity is affected because at times they don't come to work. They are not sick themselves but the spouse is in hospital on and off. Also, financially you see them going down. They take loans because some ailments are excluded in the medical scheme. And they really suffer...we are understanding. Unfortunately one of them was retrenched last year, which was very sad... (Mrs Mwala, HG).

Mrs Mwala was more reflective about individuals' experiences in comparison to the general masculine picture drawn by male managers. For example, she noted: "There are two ladies we know...we had a staff member whose spouse had that problem ... and they really suffered...which was sad". The 'masculinity' in universities is also noted by Currie et al. (2002) who argue that the impact of having more women managers can have a positive effect on introducing values and increasing collaboration and that universities need to acknowledge the personal lives and responsibilities of their workers (see also Chapter Six).

Responses to HIV and AIDS

Prevention responses have been inadequate and generally ineffective. In the poor world, the spread of HIV continues, requiring planning for increased care needs and other aspects of impact mitigation. There are few signs that this is happening (Barnett and Whiteside, 2002: 316).

Barnett and Whiteside (2002) argue that, politicians, policy makers, academics, researchers and the media, in what they refer to as 'poor world', appear to have preferred to ignore and deny the problem of HIV and AIDS. They note the lack of consideration of the potential consequences of the epidemic and what should be done about it. Their (ibid.) argument may be outdated given that their book was published in 2002 and issues of HIV and AIDS have been changing rather rapidly. However, the response to HIV and AIDS in Weruini and Holy Ghost Universities appeared to reflect what these authors refer to as a 'full measure of denial' (p. 5).

Many responses to HIV and AIDS taken by 'poor' countries rarely consider issues beyond the clinical impact of the pandemic (Barnett and Whiteside, 2002). Yet, as discussed in Chapter Seven, HIV and AIDS affects not only the health of individuals, but also their welfare and well-being.

In the interviews with the managers, I asked them what their university was doing regarding the various challenges presented by the AIDS pandemic to their staff members. Dr. Oduor, the ACU director in Weruini, said:

I cannot say we have a very consistent programme for staff. Occasionally we get antiretroviral drugs (ARVs) from the ministry of health but the supply is not regular at all. In fact, there are those who initially start the medication, then they run out of stock. Right now, as we speak, there are no ARVs in the unit...In short, we have the ARVs but not in regular supply. The main challenge here is lack of finances; it is our major drawback.

Antiretroviral treatment has brought some hope to people infected with HIV and those who have access to them are now living longer and better lives (Lindow, 2006; UNAIDS, 2005).

There has been progress in many parts of the world following access to this treatment for those who need it, not only in the rich countries of Western Europe and North America, but also a country like Botswana which has for been providing ARVs to all those who need them since 2005. The success of Antiretroviral Therapy is dependent on proper adherence levels, ensured by continuous supply of ARVs and monitoring of how the drugs are working. Short of this kind of monitoring, resistance levels increase (Barnett and Whiteside, 2002). It also helps if the people under treatment are monitored in one clinic for consistency.

If infected people can be assured that treatment will be provided, then more people may be willing to establish their HIV status as noted by UNAIDS (2005):

> Evidence and experience show that rapidly increasing availability of antiretroviral therapy leads to greater uptake of HIV testing. Kenya, for example, has seen a dramatic increase in testing and counselling uptake in 2000-2004...In Uganda, a counselling and testing clinic that had been forced to close due to lack of clients, reopened in 2002 when an antiretroviral treatment programme began... (UNAIDS, 2005: 8).

Successful treatment programmes have been seen to create a more effective environment for HIV prevention, whereas intensified prevention is needed to make HIV treatment affordable and sustainable (UNAIDS, 2005). Universities too have a responsibility to source for funds that would help make sustainable treatment available. The University of Zambia, for example, offers free ARVs to staff and their immediate dependants (Rossouw, 2005), an initiative funded by the US Government. Kenyan universities could also access this kind of help either from within the country or from outside to intensify treatment, prevention, care and support programmes for their staff. However, such help requires that those given the responsibilities to work with AIDS programmes are committed to tackling other underlying factors that fuel the spread of AIDS. These include social inequalities, stigma and denial (Barnett and Whiteside, 2002).

Similarly, in a UNAIDS report, it is noted that success of AIDS treatment requires "overcoming the existing serious barriers to access to drugs, that take the form of stigma, discrimination, gender inequality, and other human violations" (UNAIDS, 2005: 5). The findings of my study suggest that such barriers were yet to be overcome at Weruini University. In Holy Ghost, treatment was not even mentioned. This was because the position taken by management was that they did not have staff that was infected (see Chapters Four and Eight).

On the question about the responses that Weruini had taken, especially focusing on staff, the Vice Chancellor said:

> Every year we have an HIV counselling and testing day. This year it was very successful. Many people have come out to be tested and counselled...As for staff, they are adults and they have to decide if they want to access the services that we offer here. We are encouraging it... we also provide the ARVs for those who are sick and give permission to those who need to look after their relatives. The other thing is that we have a guidance and counselling centre where we talk to those who are depressed (VC, Weruini).

The Vice Chancellor noted that people were free to access HIV and AIDS services if they wished to. However, my interviews with the women had revealed that such were not actually available. The VC seems not to have taken an interest to establish exactly what was happening to his staff. For example, the ARVs were irregular and the counselling centre was almost non-existent. His attitude implied a leadership culture where the institution did not go out of its way to make sure that its staff members were coping with private challenges. The implication of such a culture on women staff was shown by the struggles of the women in this study.

In their work on the experiences of men and women academics, Currie et al. (2002) note that universities need to acknowledge the personal lives and responsibilities of their workers. The attitude of the VC reflects Barnett and Whiteside's (2002) observation that few leaders, especially in 'poor' countries, have considered the potential consequences of the epidemic and what should be done about them. The impact of HIV and AIDS on senior staff may not have as yet become very apparent to the leadership of Weruini. This could have led to the attitude of the VC that "if it is hard to see things, it is easier to deny them" (Barnett and Whiteside, 2002: 7).

The impact that the women in Weruini narrated (see Chapter Seven) would be hard to see unless one looked for it. It is not easy to measure relationships, care responsibilities, emotional stress, pain of loss and related issues that were found to be important to the women. Responding to issues that are hard to measure or see, as with the women's experiences which form the discussion of this book, requires a commitment to make the 'personal as political'.

Another interviewee, a male manager at Weruini, also referred to the counselling centre mentioned by the Vice Chancellor. This counselling centre that was talked about by these two male managers was not mentioned by any of the women in Weruini as a place where they went for any services. The fact that none of the women used these services could mean that they do not cater for the needs of senior staff members, whether affected or even probably infected.

On hearing about this service, I decided to visit it and see what was going on there. The counselling centre was part of the university clinic. I learnt from the nurses that it is a voluntary counselling and testing (VCT) clinic that was mainly serving students and support staff. I did not manage to meet the counsellor even though I went there several times.

One of the women I interviewed after I learnt about this centre commented:

> In this university, people say that in our clinic there is no confidentiality so they shy away from seeking any services there. One may fear to go there even for a simple gynaecological problem like thrush. I prefer to

go to a private doctor even if drugs are here. There is need for some work ethics, issues to do with confidentiality are necessary. One of the reasons people don't talk is because they fear. I am informing you that even myself I have no confidence to go for an HIV test here because my results will be publicised. Those are some of the things that institutions need to address (Dr. Kaiga, Senior Lecturer, Weruini).

Dr. Kaiga and other women from the two universities raised issues that were 'women specific'. The male professors may not even have thought about a problem like thrush that affects many women. In a university where the majority of those in senior policy making positions are male, it may be difficult for such women's issues to be taken into consideration.

It is common practice in universities that it is the professors who make decisions. They head departments, represent the university to the government, serve on many boards and make all other important decisions (Acker, 1994). In a university which had only eight women professors and associate professors compared with 36 men professors and associates, women's issues may not get priority. The fewer women there are at the top, the fewer they are in committees that make decisions. These few women generally become silenced (Currie et al., 2002; Onsongo, 2005).

The health centre in Holy Ghost was also said to be similar to that of Weruini:

The problem with our services is lack of confidentiality. There is that fear that what if I talk to so and so and what if the news will come out ... let me shock you. Recently, I went to the clinic in campus and the doctor was telling me: 'I have seen so many people with STDs'. You know, I felt ouch! What if I was coming with a sexually transmitted disease (STD)? I would have just walked away. In such a place (clinic) you can get records of people who have been seen in a particular day and you can even follow up a little bit and find out that they might have come for an HIV test. So it puts you off (Ms. Mugasia, Lecturer, HG).

Issues dealing with sexuality are more sensitive where women are concerned as I discuss in Chapter Nine. It would be difficult for women to talk about sexually-related problems, even common ones like thrush, which Dr. Kaiga and Ms Mugasia mentioned, much less the more stigmatised HIV and AIDS, and in a clinic where ethical issues are not taken seriously.

Several women said they did not know what the university was doing to support staff that were either infected or affected. Dr. Wangare said that she had attended an AIDS workshop for senior managers at Weruini. The issues discussed in that workshop, according to Dr. Wangare, "did not reach a deeper and critical level ...reflecting on how they fit in the bigger picture". Some of the issues that require more critical analysis could be related to gender and sexuality. The present study was meant to provide a possible beginning for thinking 'deeper and critically'. This was shown by the number of women respondents who commented at the end of the interviews that they had not thought about AIDS in ways that this study made them think. Others hoped that the findings of my study could be used as a beginning for more 'talking' about the issues that mattered to them as women, as noted in the following excerpt:

> There is something missing in Weruini, which was different in the university where I did my PhD in the UK. In that University there was some concern for those small things that matter to women. I had just registered and had my two year-old baby in the crèche, and then there I was and I got pregnant again. Oh my God, I was so shocked – and I went to my supervisor and told her – Oh I don't know what to do but I am pregnant – I was afraid I could lose my registration. And she told me 'you can take a year off' ... and I was like, 'is that possible? You mean I can take a year off and not lose my registration'? And she told me 'oh sure you need to take care of yourself and the baby and then you can have both of them at the crèche'. Looking at Weruini now I can see – we require policies in our universities that cater for women's unique needs. My one fear is that many of these men will think such issues are trivial and are not the university business and they should be sorted out at home. I hope this study will be a beginning for better things to come (Gaudencia, Lecturer, Weruini).

Here, Gaudencia is reflecting on her university where women's roles (in this case reproductive) were recognised and validated. Western universities, like the one Gaudencia was referring to, appear to have different cultures, seemingly more accommodating to women's issues. Even though studies have also shown that women are also disadvantaged in the UK universities, some facilities like crèche are common unlike the situation in Kenya. My own experience studying in a UK university has also shown that there is some room for discussing personal problems, at least for students. However, just like this study found to be happening in Weruini and Holy Ghost, female staff in UK universities also have to deal with challenges that are purely related to gender (see later in this chapter).

The data so far suggests that neither Weruini nor Holy Ghost had taken account of gender issues in their responses to HIV and AIDS. However, there were differences in their responses. At Holy Ghost, some women claimed that there was some discrimination against staff who were suspected or known to be infected:

> During the university restructuring recently, four of our staff that were retrenched were feared to be HIV positive. You see we had this blood donation day and the HIV results were revealed to the administration. It was shocking when people discovered their HIV status ...it also came out that there was a lot of sexual activity among students and staff, and staff with staff. Two drivers and two librarians were said to have been HIV infected and they were all retrenched. One of the drivers died soon after he was retrenched. A woman senior librarian also died within a month after losing her job. From that incident we came up with a two-day training for staff. But as long as people distance themselves from HIV, the training may not have any impact (Ms. Mueni, Lecturer HG).

According to Ms Mueni, Holy Ghost had already reacted by sponsoring an HIV and AIDS training programme for staff, on realising that some people were infected. However, Ms Mueni noted that even though there was this training, her colleagues still distanced themselves from the problem of AIDS. Barnett and Whiteside (2002) note this distancing of academia and policy makers (in Africa) from the effects of HIV and AIDS:

> There has been a full measure of denial. Some, perhaps the majority seeing no way to engage with what has appeared to be an overwhelming problem...others fear the pandemic stigma may besmirch their professional lives (p. 5).

In Holy Ghost, this distancing could be due to fear that they could lose their jobs if discovered, just like their colleagues. There was also an underlying fear among staff that if they appeared concerned about AIDS issues, they may be mistaken for being sexually immoral. (Christianity and its approach to HIV and AIDS as a disease of immorality are discussed at length in Chapter Nine.) Besides the direct discrimination of staff found to be infected as mentioned by some of the women in Holy Ghost, the responses in the two universities reflected an attitude of "if it is difficult to see what is happening, harder to measure, easiest to deny" (Barnett and Whiteside, 2002: 5). Such an attitude is likely to be more damaging to women than men, because women are likely to be involved in activities that are more difficult to measure.

Weruini University AIDS Policy: Any Gender Issues?

In this section, I look at whether the AIDS policy acknowledges that men and women require different policy responses given the existing gender roles and responsibilities in Kenya. The AIDS policy in Weruini University was finalised in 2003. It touches on various aspects of the university including students, staff and the curriculum. I only focus on those areas relevant to my research question: whether the policy considers women's experiences.

In the introduction, the policy states:

> The HIV and AIDS pandemic has affected Weruini University in various ways; there has, for instance, been a significant loss of workplace cohesion due to low morale, absenteeism and high recruitment and

medical expenses. The university is also losing trained personnel and students, thereby affecting graduate output and manpower. The university has shown various responses to HIV and AIDS in order to curb the pandemic in the institution (Weruini AIDS policy, 2003).

The introduction is gender neutral. From this extract, one would think that some initiatives have been taken, especially to deal with staff morale. However, the findings of this study suggest that nothing has been done that reaches the women who were affected and probably infected.

One of the challenges facing AIDS initiatives is that many people do not yet know whether they are infected (UNAIDS, 2005). As I mentioned in Chapter One, I did not ask the women if they were infected, but many of the women told me that they had not been tested for HIV. Some said they feared a positive result, while others said they would be uncomfortable to visit a VCT in case they met people who knew them. Mrs Wandera was especially concerned about meeting any of her current or even former students at a VCT. During our conversation over lunch, she asked me whether I knew of a VCT where she would be sure not to meet people she knew. She was keen to know if I had gone for a test and where. I told her that I was lucky to have been tested in London where I was unlikely to meet people I knew. This was an indication of the stigma that still surrounds HIV and AIDS.

AIDS-related stigma appears very difficult to remove as the literature indicates (Barnett and Whiteside, 2002; Ciambrone, 2003; Green, 1996; Hunter, 2003; Manchester, 2001; Mbilinyi and Kaihula, 2000; O'Sullivan, 1996; Parker and Aggleton, 2003; Wood, 2002). This is because HIV and AIDS "mixes sex, death and fear of disease" (Barnett and Whiteside, 2002: 66). In Chapter Nine sex, silence and stigma are further explored looking at their contribution to the denial and inaction in the universities.

None of the 'various responses' mentioned in the policy include making the university environment more supportive to women's needs, where they can find comfort and safety to talk about such matters that cause fear and anxiety (see section Chapter

Seven). Two women interviewees at Weruini, said they found the university "very matter of fact", something that made them feel uncomfortable about the place, as they describe in some of the following excerpts:

> There are no support systems that the university has provided. Here I stand to be corrected since I may be the only one who is not aware. Probably, the administration has done something for staff that I am not aware of, but what I know they have put in place targets students. They think that they can fight the AIDS epidemic more from the students' perspective because it is at that level where they have put in place programmes like 'ICL' where students meet and they talk in a place they find safe. My daughter is a student here and says they are very happy with ICL... The too matter of fact attitude as far as staff members are concerned is something that worries me (Mrs Bihanya, Lecturer, Weruini).

> When I talk of the university, I feel in many ways it is not a friendly place; it is not a place one feels comfortable. I find people stick to themselves, are secretive and always official. It's always that habit of 'how are you?' Nobody tries to chat with anybody and considering there is no forum for it, we do not even have a common place where we can have tea as a department. ...it is different in the corporate world where I have worked before where people tend to work more in teams. The problem with the university is that we always come and go and we never meet. I have an office here but I've never sat here for more than four hours (Mrs Munyi, Lecturer Weruini).

These two women concur that the culture in their university left little room for people to express and talk about their personal issues. In their study, Currie et al. (2002) make similar observations to Mrs Munyi and Mrs Bihanya. They observe that women favour a consultative, collaborative approach, which encourages people to work in teams. However, the university culture is based on competition rather than cooperation, and authority rather than collegial support. This masculine culture may lead to increased staff exhaustion and stress, especially to women who have more family responsibilities compared to men (Currie et al., 2002).

The Weruini AIDS policy seems to have taken on board personal issues of staff as stated in the specific objectives of the policy that focus on the staff welfare:

This policy aims at promoting HIV and AIDS education for employees' families; all our operations to have clearly defined policies and procedures, which will reflect local practices, procedures, culture and legislation; discourage workplace stigmatisation and discrimination against those living with HIV (Weruini AIDS policy, 2003).

Although these objectives appear to be considerate of the private needs of employees, the problem lies on lack of programmes that reflect what is on paper. None of the 10 women from Weruini said that they had heard of any training about HIV and AIDS that had particularly targeted their families. They all said that they were unaware of anything that was targeting staff members, much less their families. For example, Prof. Nyaboke, who was also a dean, noted:

We have an AIDS policy. I don't know whether you've heard about it. I think it was a move in the right direction, but I wonder how many people are actually aware that it exists. Maybe I am aware because of where I sit. The students have their own movements like ICL and peer counselling, which are doing a good job. I really don't know whether there is anything going on among the staff. We have participated but seeing how heavy this thing is, I think more needs to be done, and especially on issues like those we have talked about here. I have never given them much thought, but I know they matter (Prof Nyaboke, Weruini).

Prof. Nyaboke's sentiments indicate that having a policy written is one thing, while having it implemented and touching on what really concerns all people is another. The picture given to the public differs from the reality on the ground. Prof. Nyaboke gave an example of a woman support staff in her office who had died of AIDS-related complications. When she became dean, she found the woman unwell. She said that having experienced her sister in law's sickness (who later died of AIDS), she supported the ailing woman until her final days. She allowed her to take days off and gave her a lighter workload. However, Nyaboke noted that this kind of response that depends on an individual is not sustainable. Thus, the institution needs to design responses that reach out to all staff members regardless of their position or who they report to.

Prof. Nyaboke also mentioned the students' movement of 'I Choose Life' (ICL), which I introduced in Chapter Three and discuss at length in the present chapter. The model used by ICL appeared very practical and one would wish it could be used for staff.

In the section about care and support, the policy states that Weruini will seek to:

> Help those who are uninfected to remain free from infection; provide HIV and AIDS counselling; create an environment where people living with HIV and AIDS are safe to reveal their status and seek appropriate support and counselling; ensure that all records connected with the counselling and support services are kept confidential...; equip the university community with skills that will enable them to live and work in societies with increasing rates of HIV infection; provide care for those infected and affected by HIV and AIDS; provide support groups for staff with HIV and AIDS and for their families and colleagues (Weruini AIDS policy 2003).

As I have pointed out so far, none of the women were aware of any of these services that are mentioned here. Dr. Kaiga (quoted earlier in this chapter), for example, said that the clinical support lacked qualified staff who could treat medical information with confidentiality. In the above quoted statement, it is mentioned that Weruini would provide care and support for those affected by HIV and AIDS. All the 10 women from Weruini university were affected by HIV/AIDS, yet none of them had received the mentioned support. Nor were they aware what support existed. Apart from Dr. Wangare, a head of department, and Prof. Nyaboke, a dean, who were aware of this policy, none of the other women were even sure if there was a policy.

I later learnt that there had been a lot of pressure from the Commission for Higher Education (CHE) for universities to write AIDS policies. Many of these documents were almost being duplicated from those drafted earlier, with no serious thought being given to their implementation. This made me understand the reasons why there was such a disconnection between the policy at Weruini and the practice. I also learnt that ACUs were also established under similar pressure, and not surprisingly many of them were not operational (Nyutho et al., 2005).

Writing about issues of sexual harassment in Southern African universities, Bennet (2005) notes that university policies that are written without intricate theorising and strategising by people who truly understand the issues, rarely have the desired impact. Such policies usually leave huge gaps between what is avowed and what is met in practice (Bennet, 2005). This was the situation in Weruini and is likely to be replicated in other universities in Kenya in their rush to write policies without "engaging with complex climates of diversity, discrimination, opportunity and change by which all current higher education institutions can be characterized" (Bennet, 2005: 6).

If policies are framed within a typical male perspective, even though they may sound 'women-friendly', the actual implementation becomes gender blind, as seen in Weruini AIDS policy. The policy appears inclusive to an outsider, yet in reality it has not been translated into programmes from which women can benefit. In male-dominated organisations like universities, women's personal problems tend to be viewed as a sign of weakness even though they bear no relation to the intellectual abilities that the women possess (Coate, 1999). As a result, women may not feel comfortable to ask for the inclusion of personal issues into university HIV and AIDS policies and programmes, because they may be seen as unrelated to the work situation.

The policy states that, "The University will provide support groups for staff with HIV and AIDS and for their families and colleagues". However, the women interviewed were not aware of any support network that they could join. Neither had they heard of any initiative to set up such a network. The support that many women mentioned as helpful came from their churches, families and friends from outside the university, an issue I explore further in the following section.

Universities' Support for Students vis-à-vis Academic Women

As I have indicated earlier in the present chapter, the support for senior women staff appeared to be lacking in both Weruini and Holy Ghost Universities. Throughout the research, I noted the number of times students were mentioned, both by management and by the women interviewed. It seems that universities are almost exclusively concerned with the welfare of students.

Research about academic women has shown that they are usually expected to provide support especially to students, yet they tend to receive little support from the institutions themselves (Deem, 2003; Morley, 1999; Probert, 2005). Women, therefore, are faced with the challenges of providing support not only in their personal roles, but also at professional levels. And yet none of these sets of support-giving is recognised as 'work.'

Morley (2003b), in her study of academic women's experiences, found that women academics were expected to provide extra support to students more than men. This was especially more demanding given the huge increase of student numbers and workload in UK higher education, coupled with demands to undertake more research and publishing. The extra demands on women to provide support to students not only for students' academic work, but also for their personal problems, were mentioned by some of the women in my study:

> Students normally come to me for counselling. Recently I had a very complicated case and because the mother is my friend, I thought I could not handle it. The mother has booked an appointment to see me and the son has agreed to open up to the mother...The mother is upcountry and the son comes to see me so the last time I realised he was very depressed and I referred him to our students' counselling centre (Mrs Wandera, Lecturer, HG).

I normally counsel students who come to me with problems. I had one with a very complicated case. He was mentally disturbed as he was hallucinating that some people wanted to kill him. I talked to him about Christ and he got saved. Now he prays when such hallucinations come. He later came back to me and told me that he no longer needed medication as prayers were working (Mrs Wakaba, Lecturer, HG).

Many women supported students without complaining, although they commented that they had a lot of work to do. This finding concurs with Probert's study (2005) where it was found that women academics spend more time than do men on student welfare and pastoral work. In Probert's study, 42.6 per cent of women spent time on student welfare work compared to 26.5 per cent men, while 27.8 per cent of women spent time mentoring students compared to 17.6 per cent of men.

In relation to HIV and AIDS, students in both Weruini and Holy Ghost Universities seemed to be getting some good support. In one of my early field visits to Holy Ghost, I visited the 'I Choose Life' (ICL) office where I spoke to the deputy project officer (see Chapter Three for an introduction to ICL). A resource like ICL did not exist for staff. The ICL offices were well organised in both universities. They looked welcoming and 'youth-friendly'. On the day of my visit to the Holy Ghost ICL offices, the students were busy planning for an upcoming peer counsellors' training. They were also coordinating a mobile VCT that was based in campus at the time. I visited this VCT and found a long queue of students waiting to be tested (from my field notes).

Several of the interviewees mentioned the emphasis on students as far as AIDS responses were concerned:

For the last two years, we have been training students on HIV and AIDS. We train about 300 students every semester and they graduate formally. We invite people from CHE to come and talk to them. Another thing I've done is to form HIV and AIDS associations among students. I've tried to convert the traditional district focus associations into HIV and AIDS associations... (Dr Oduor, ACU Director, Weruini).

The ACU initiative was set up with students in mind since, as you know, a lot of sexual activity has to do with peer pressure...Through the ACU, there was an aggressive campaign to popularise the use of condoms so that various points in the hostels and the various resident houses have buckets of condoms at strategic places (Prof Atwoli, ACU board, Weruini).

I find the peer counselling education very important because it is the initiative we have taken very seriously. We have trained several peer counsellors among the students.... We also have the university counsellors who get involved in what is going on and who become aware of the forms of counselling that are appropriate for the purpose of stemming the spread of this scourge... We have trained quite a large number so that we have more students who are trained and I believe that a peer counsellor is himself benefiting from that information (Dr Kivuu, ACU director, HG).

The statements quoted above suggest that support for students in respect of HIV and AIDS related issues was fairly adequate in both universities. Two reasons can be advanced for this emphasis on students, while excluding staff. One, as noted earlier, there is still a stereotype belief that more educated and probably older people know already enough about AIDS, and they are less at risk, so they do not require as much attention as young people. Second, there is increased competition to attract students, especially among the private universities, and partly the self-sponsored programmes within the public universities, thereby neglecting staff interests. The self-sponsored programmes, which are popularly referred to as 'parallel programmes', have been established in public universities to cater for students not absorbed in the 'regular' intakes. The students taken in these programmes normally pay tuition for themselves, unlike the regular ones who mainly access government loans. The parallel tuition fees are equivalent to that in private universities and therefore these programmes have become an important avenue for income generation in public universities. My experience in teaching in one such parallel programme showed that these groups of students are treated much better than the regulars as lecturers are keen to maintain large classes because the pay is linked to the numbers.

The financial crisis facing African academics is an issue that has been noted by others (Lindow, 2006; Teferra and Altbach, 2004). With the fast expanding university sector in Kenya, there is competition amongst universities (Teferra and Altbach, 2004). The Commission for Higher Education has also become more vigilant with the private universities because there have been some concerns about the quality of degrees being offered in these new universities. Whereas these quality checks are good for students who stand to get better value for their money, there is the question, which Morley (2003a: ix) poses: "I question whether quality assurance procedures are producing new systems of power and reinforcing gendered power relations in the academy". I too question if all is well in universities where gendered division of labour persists, in a similar way to the one Morley (2003a) describes in Britain. Increased staff gender imbalances in African universities have also been noted by Teferra and Altbach (2004).

In Chapter Seven, I have noted that the women I spoke to receive little support from the universities. Besides the expectation to provide non-academic support to students, one of the senior lecturers at Holy Ghost also talked about the long hours of teaching she had to work, which, coupled with family responsibilities, made it almost impossible for her to complete her PhD proposal. She was almost giving up on the studies, as she was already 60 years old. This is the same woman who had earlier discussed how the illness of her mother-in-law had affected her work, as she spent a lot of time looking after her:

> Here we have to do 12 hours of teaching and in each class I have about 200 students, the classes are very big. My classes are very popular so most students come to them. Like you can see, these are the lists of the students I have. So I find myself teaching and marking throughout the week. But let me tell you what can happen; if one is very keen she can embark on a PhD and then if the proposal is ready, one is allocated only two classes instead of four. At the stage of data collection, the

university could give one leave for one semester to allow the staff member work better ...the university encourages studies but you know you have to start off and you know a proposal takes a lot of time. When you go and show what you have done, you will be given time off, so one cannot say the university is preventing us, we just need to work harder (Mrs Wakaba, Lecturer, HG).

Based on what the women said, one can argue that it may be easier for a man to complete his PhD proposal and then get time off to carry out his research. Women in this study talked about their gender roles like care for the ill and other domestic responsibilities, which affected their academic work (see also Currie et al., 2002). Their male partners on the other hand could concentrate with their work without many domestic interruptions (see Chapter Six and also noted in my field notes as many women mentioned it during our discussions after the interview). Mrs Wakaba did not see any problem with the university regulations, which treated men and women the same way. However, interviews with the women in this study suggest that there are times when it would be helpful to treat men and women differently, where their needs and circumstances differ. Mrs Wakaba believed that all she needed to do was to work extra hard so that she could complete her proposal and earn her time off. In a way she blamed herself for not working hard enough to complete her proposal. The strategy of women working extra hard in order to survive in the academy has been documented in other studies (e.g., Mabokela, 2003; Onsongo, 2005; Wyn et al., 2000).

In Weruini (a public university) the situation was slightly different, where competition to attract students may not have been as high as in Holy Ghost. However, classes in public universities can be very large (even over 500 students), especially in Years One and Two (I observed the size of classes while at these universities). Lower classes tend to be allocated to junior academics (lecturers and below), the majority of whom are women. Prof. Atwoli of Weruini, for example, told me that he normally taught only one Masters' degree class every semester, which takes only three hours per week (noted in the field diary as this was said after the interview). It is not surprising therefore that Prof. Atwoli has a long list of publications (He showed me the latest one that was about to be launched).

Men and women respondents mentioned lack of finance as the cause of poor AIDS services, especially for staff members. The financing of non-academic programmes, which are viewed as not directly benefiting students, is a challenge facing many Kenyan universities (CHE and UNESCO, 2004). Generally, projects that address the private lives of staff members tend to receive the least priority. Women tend to be more affected by private challenges as findings of this study suggest. Unfortunately, women's issues usually receive the least attention, especially where there is scarcity of resources.

On this, Fogelberg et al. (1999), writing about universities in Finland, note that addressing gender equality is hard work, yet it is work that "still remains unseen, unacknowledged and performed with minimum resources" (p. 11). The situation in Kenyan universities is likely to be worse given the lack of interest in gender issues from top management, who happen to be mainly men, as this study has indicated.

Summary and Conclusion

My discussion in the present chapter indicates that nothing is being done in the two universities to support the senior women staff members whom I spoke to. In relation to gender issues, the responses are at best gender-neutral but mainly gender-blind. These two universities are taking few tangible steps to help staff members to cope with HIV and AIDS. Holy Ghost seems to be discriminating against staff infected with the HIV virus, thus making it more difficult for other staff to talk about their own experiences. This study suggests that the few responses that were made to tackle HIV and AIDS staff challenges were random rather than systematic.

The involvement of senior staff in HIV and AIDS responses appears to be indiscernible. The universities' main concern seems to focus on students. The AIDS policy at Weruini University lacks in the actual implementation of what it proposes. Given the gap between what is stated in the policy and what is actually practised, it is imperative that there should be a re-conceptualisation of the terms and conditions under which issues of gender inequity, access to social presence and power are predicated and addressed to. This would include accepting, as necessary, the inclusion of the private sphere in public policy, challenging gender roles and interrogating issues of access to voice.

To conclude this chapter, I find Bennet's (2005) assertion relevant regarding policies on sexual harassment in higher education concerning issues that lie within the private sphere:

> The process of policy implementation is notoriously vulnerable to the complexities of 'deep culture' within institutional life – those vectors, and forces, of power formation not usually visible at the formal surface of the institutional structure (p. 22).

In the case of policies on HIV and AIDS, for example, there is an interconnection between issues of sexuality, silence, stigma, traditions, religion and gender inequality – all of which interlock to create a difficult terrain for any meaningful and strategic intervention. Chapter Nine further explores these issues.

= 9

Sexuality, Silence and Stigma

AIDS touches off deeply buried fears of ignorance of sex...
AIDS has opened up space and legitimised a feminist discussion
on sexuality...
O'Sullivan (1996: 168)

Introduction

Sexuality is intricately linked to practically every aspect of people's lives; from pleasure, power, politics and recreation, to disease, violence and war, among others (Tamale, 2005). One of the factors that have been found to be driving HIV and AIDS stigma is its sexual nature (Campbell et al., 2006). The present chapter explores how the discourses of sexuality among my respondents could increase our understanding of the responses (discussed in the previous chapter) to HIV and AIDS in the two Universities. In this chapter, I address the research question: How did sexuality-related stigma contribute to the inaction and silence about HIV and AIDS amongst university staff (especially among senior women)?

This research question is answered by exploring the underlying explanations that link sexuality in Kenya to shame, silence and stigma, particularly among highly educated people. I focus my argument on how colonialism and Christianity could have contributed to the current discourses of shame and stigma associated with sex. I then discuss ways in which fear of being identified with a stigmatised disease leads to silence about AIDS in the two universities. My focus is on heterosexuality because none of the respondents in my study mentioned or even implied that they had homosexual or other forms of sexual tendencies. I focus on heterosexuality because it was the only form of sexuality that the women referred to given that it has been treated as more legitimate than any other form of sexuality in many African cultures. Heterosexuality is usually justified from a religio-cultural perspective (Arnfred, 2004; Becker, 2004; Machera, 2004; McFadden, 2003).

Background to Sex-Related Shame and Stigma in Kenya

To understand the complexity of HIV and AIDS, I found it worthwhile to look at some historical background to current attitudes about sexuality in Africa. This is because my study was carried out against a backdrop of multiple patriarchies and the legacy of colonialism. Hunter (2003) provides a background to the origins of the shame that became associated with sex in Africa long before AIDS was reported noting that during the colonial times, the British set up laws in the colonies that were tougher than those in their own country because they believed that 'primitive' practices required harsher enforcement" (p. 168). Similarly, Tamale (2005) notes that, "Africans were encouraged to reject their previous beliefs and values to adopt the 'civilised ways' of the colonial masters" (p.11). In colonial days, according to Hunter (2003):

> Victorians thought that tropical climates acted as breeding grounds for disease, inflamed passions and negated reason ... primitive peoples, they believed, were simply more tolerant of filth and STDs because of their unrestrained sexuality, both symptoms of non-western and moral decay (p.169).

The colonialist overlords viewed Africans as having wild sexual habits that needed to be controlled (Becker, 2004; Elkins, 2005). To some European colonialists, "African sexuality was especially dark, primitive, uncontrolled and excessive..." (Hunter, 2003: 170). But Hunter argues that there were some colonialists who thought that African sexuality had worsened because of colonial rule. The colonialists, holding the latter view, thought that Christianity had destroyed indigenous moral systems, displacing traditionally severe punishments for sexual offences, even though they had not replaced them with other systems of social control.

In spite of the two different views on African sexuality, the advocates of both views concurred that "Africans and their sexuality were savage" (Becker, 2004: 37). The colonisers were on a "civilising mission" (Elkins, 2005: 116). This 'mission' led to a breakdown of many traditional practices where sexual matters were handled (Ahlberg, 1991; Kenyatta, 1938).

In the absence of traditional systems where sexual matters were addressed, many Kenyan cultures still view as taboo talking about sex in public where people of different age groups, gender and ethnicity are mixed. This has brought about confusion as far as sex education is concerned. Parents no longer have places to take their children for education on sexuality and the church is unclear about ways of teaching it, given the shame that has become associated with the subject often originating from the colonial era.

A senior lecturer at Weruini University told me:

> I've always said that it is unfortunate that for us, African people. Christianity, colonialism and even modern education interfered with the cultural ways of discussing sex issues. Some people have grown up with an African cultural background where sex is not something that is discussed anywhere. It is discussed among age-mates but you see again, this is a very multi-ethnic community and each ethnic group has its own way of discussing sex issues. One place where colleagues can freely talk about sex matters here is at the club where people go to drink and talk politics. These are not necessarily networks for friends, but just a drinking place... women rarely go to the Weruini Club, for example, unless accompanied by their husbands. If they go alone, they can be mistaken for something else (Dr Kaiga, Senior Lecturer Weruini).

Dr. Kaiga noted that social places like the university club could present suitable space where people could freely interact and discuss issues that would otherwise not come up in the office. However, as a woman, she did not feel comfortable in such a place.

She noted that women who frequented the club might be seen to be of loose morals.

Dr. Kaiga also mentioned that the contexts where sex was discussed traditionally have changed over the years. Whereas in the past there were special times and places – for example, initiation and wedding ceremonies where sexual matters would be discussed – these days such talk has been left to beer drinking places (dominated by men). The modern Western culture, though more open about sex compared to the African culture, demonises it more (Becker, 2004; Foucault, 1978). These contradictory discourses on sexuality have contributed to the shaping of sexual values and beliefs amongst many 'modern' Kenyans. The spaces where sexual issues may be discussed tend to be dominated by men. Among several communities in Kenya, male circumcision is still an important occasion where men talk about sexuality (Nelson, 1987).

Moreover, in many African cultures, the subject of sexuality seems to have been handled with great care and there was less stigma and shame linked to it (Arnfred, 2004; Becker, 2004; McFadden, 2003; Mufune, 2003; Pereira, 2003; Tamale, 2005). Pereira (2003: 62), for example, notes that the notion of sexuality as 'bad' or 'filthy' is relatively new in Africa because it was introduced to Africans through colonialism and Christianity. Among the Agikuyu, for example, there were restrictions on sex before marriage for both men and women (Kenyatta, 1938). Training on sexual matters was offered to both boys and girls before they were initiated (Ahlberg, 1991; Kenyatta, 1938). Kenyatta writes about a practice that was known as ngwiko (a form of foreplay). Young people used ngwiko to express their sexuality without penetration. During ngwiko, the couple would share an intimate encounter, with the woman's skirt tightly tied to her thighs to avoid possible penetration. Furthermore, the practice of a number of men and women having ngwiko in one room was common. This enhanced the peer pressure and minimised chances of full sexual intercourse (Ahlberg, 1991), while still providing young people with a chance to experience sexual pleasure.

According to Kenyatta (1938) missionaries misunderstood *ngwiko*, branding it sinful and anyone caught performing it would be punished. Hence much of the stigma that is currently associated with sex (at least among the Agikuyu) can be linked to colonialism and Christianity. The Gikuyu people's way of life was the most disrupted by colonial rule in Kenya (Elkins, 2005). In addition, the modern subordinate status of women in sexual relationships among the Gikuyu can be linked to the stigma that Christianity associated with sex. This is because women found it difficult to talk about sex even with their husbands, otherwise they would appear 'unschooled' and 'backward' (Arnfred, 2004).

Besides *ngwiko*, the colonialists and the missionaries mistook clitoridectomy as an evil and backward practice, without providing any alternative for the important role it played in initiating girls into womanhood. According to Kenyatta (1938), African communities that practised clitoridectomy performed the act "to symbolically represent the flow of life through the shedding of blood from the organs of reproduction" (p. 98). While I do not support clitoridectomy, I argue that during this initiation ritual, women had a chance to express their sexuality without shame or fear, as they educated the initiates.

Similarly, Mbiti (1975) a leading writer on African traditional religions, does not mention anywhere that sex was viewed as an act of shame. Rather, he notes that the sexual act was not viewed as immoral because it was normally performed within the rules of many of the African communities.

The AmaZulu of South Africa had initiation schools for young men and women. In these schools, young people were taught how to prepare for adult life and the way to relate to people of the opposite sex and to have sex by stimulation and penetration was forbidden until marriage (Khathide, 2003).

Colonialists and missionaries tried to make Africans develop a sense of shame about their sexual practices as a sign of becoming 'modern and civilised'. This focus on modernity could help explain why educated people are largely silent about sexuality leading to more stigma of a disease like HIV and AIDS that is seen to be mainly heterosexually transmitted in Africa (Barnett and Whiteside, 2002).

Hunter (2003) argues that the way syphilis was handled in the colonies can now be seen as one of the causes of sex-related shame and stigma. She notes that colonialists could not quite agree on the best way to deal with the problem of syphilis for African natives. A colonial director of medical services in Uganda is quoted by Hunter (2003) to have said that:

> The local African is especially immoral or even that he is amoral but that his way of looking at sexual contact is different from what is generally accepted to be that of European Christian Civilisation (p. 172).

The medical officer cited above argued that the war had worsened the disruption of native custom and social practice initiated by colonisation. Since tradition could not be restored, colonialists believed that "a new morality had to be forged" (Hunter, 2003: 172). The officer felt that there had been a time lag between the disruption of traditional control systems and the growth of a Christian code to replace it. Colonialists had differing opinions about the best way of dealing with sexually transmitted infections (STIs), and whether quick and free treatment would solve the problem. The worry amongst the colonialists was that treating syphilis could lead to increased sexual immorality among Africans. On this, Hunter (2003) notes that the colonialists felt that, "once Africans saw that STDs could be treated, they would become even more promiscuous" (p. 174). Arnfred (2004) similarly notes that, "the icons of syphilis are no longer homeless. They have been appropriately filled up and even extended with new related icons of HIV/AIDS" (p. 67).

The shame associated with a sexually transmitted illness makes those infected or affected (especially women) feel "worthless, undesirable and uneasy about their own as well as their children's health and futures" (Ciambrone, 2003: 38). In her study, Ciambrone (2003) interviewed 37 HIV-positive women in the USA, many of whom had internalised the shame and stigma associated with HIV and AIDS. They viewed themselves as "abnormal and dirty, filthy... less of a good person...like the leprosy in the Bible" (Ciambrone, 2003: 39). From this historical background some discourses on HIV and AIDS have emerged, which I discuss in the following section.

Sex Discourses and Their Influence on Attitudes and Practice in the Two Universities

In Chapter Five, I discussed my understanding of discourse and noted that HIV and AIDS has become a discipline with its own discourse. The different layers of patriarchal structures operating within the universities, nationally and globally, inform this discourse. In this section I explore the different discourses that emerged in this study which include morality, silence, shame, stigma and blame.

The Morality Discourse

From the discussion earlier in the present chapter, I have provided one of the arguments that can be used to explain why educated Kenyans seem to find it difficult to openly declare their HIV status. Some of the women in my study also held 'moralist' views about AIDS:

> HIV and AIDS is not like cancer. The methods of contracting it are what make it shameful...and that is where the stigma is... you see, we cannot remove the society from the issue of morality. Society still expects people to be moral. The issue of morality makes the whole thing to be stigmatised (Mrs Musoga, Lecturer, Weruini).

The linking of sex with morality tends to lead to the stigmatisation of those affected by HIV and AIDS (Lindow, 2006). In the above quoted statement, Mrs Musoga felt that it would be difficult to separate morality from AIDS, because unlike a disease like cancer, which also does not have a cure, AIDS is sexually transmitted.

Issues of morality dominate the AIDS discourse where those infected are viewed as being immoral. Studies continue to show that women who get infected or affected by HIV are more stigmatised than are men as they are often perceived to be of loose morals (Ciambrone, 2003; Lipinge et al., 2004). Literature, which has focused on the experiences of infected men, especially gay white men, has shown that they too suffer stigma and discrimination.

Infected women suffer unique challenges that are not typically central concerns of their male counterparts (Ciambrone, 2003). For example, women's issues include; poverty, caring for others, reproductive decisions, access to health care and social services, negotiating condom use, feelings of undesirability, among others (Ciambrone, 2003). Similarly, Campbell et al. (2006) note that in their study of AIDS stigma in South Africa:

> A key factor sustaining stigmatisation of sexuality and HIV/AIDS was the link between sex, sin and morality. The church was the main contributor of the symbolic ammunition that sustained this link. People often referred to HIV/AIDS as God's punishment for sin and evil, linking it to Biblical prophecies about the end of the world (p. 134).

This persisting attitude that those who get AIDS have sinned or are immoral fails to consider the fact that many women in Africa have little power in their sexual relationships (Wood, 2002). In any case, those mostly affected by AIDS may not necessarily be having any more sex than those not affected. This is an issue that the dominant AIDS discourse has failed to put into consideration. Barnett and Whiteside (2002) make a similar argument:

> Sexual intercourse (of whatever variety: oral, anal, vaginal) is not intrinsically a 'risky' behaviour...However, when a deadly disease appears and the social and economic environment is such as to facilitate rapid and/or frequent partner change, then the environment may be described as a risk environment...the riskiness of the behaviour is a characteristic of the environment rather than of the individuals or the particular practices (p. 81).

Such an argument has not been popularised enough so that people can stop apportioning blame to individuals who get infected with HIV. Some churches and donors continue to pursue moral discourses that increase stigma and silence. This is especially worse for Kenyan women, who may be quite helpless as far as the control of their sexual lives is concerned or they lack 'bedroom power' (Machera, 2004: 167). This lack of bedroom power deprives many women of the right to decide if and when to have safe sex (ibid). Whereas men are given sexual freedom, women do not have the same freedom and many of them are at the mercy of their husbands or partners (Lipinge et al., 2004; Machera, 2004).

Discourse of Silence

Silence about sexuality was another issue that seemed to dominate HIV and AIDS discourse among the women I spoke to. Several women in my study said that the topic of sex was rarely discussed with their spouses and even their children. Many of them, like Mrs Musoga, as quoted earlier in this chapter, said that they only hoped and trusted that their husbands were not unfaithful.

From the interviews, it was clear that sex was not a topic that was talked about with husbands, as shown by the extract from an interview with a lecturer from Holy Ghost:

> We do not really talk about it [sex]. In a way, we may talk about general issues or if someone we know has AIDS, then we discuss it. For me I know the main method that AIDS is transmitted [sexually]. So I think about my sexual behaviour and my husband's. I am sure about my own sexual behaviour and I can also say I am almost sure about my husband's sexual behaviour. I am a Christian and he also is a Christian so I put a lot of faith in that. The rest I leave to God (Bahati, Lecturer, HG).

Many of the respondents in this study commented that the overall causes of silences that were associated with HIV and AIDS in the universities and in Kenyan society at large were the stigma and shame associated with a sexually transmitted disease. During my interviews, the issue of shame that I have discussed in this chapter was seen to have contributed to AIDS-related stigma. The following are examples of the women's views:

AIDS is a disease that even among us academia, a highly educated lot, are still very ashamed of. I think this shame is related to a very important aspect that we don't discuss, which is sex. Until we are open about sex, we cannot begin to talk about HIV and AIDS... So I must say staff are affected and I think they just don't talk about it (Dr Kaiga, Senior Lecturer, Weruini).

The other thing why there is this stigmatisation is because of the way HIV is transmitted. This has been mainly through sex or so we are made to believe. As long as it is through sexual contact, it will always be branded a sin on a religious point of view (Prof Atieno, Weruini).

We had a meeting after we buried my brother ...some of our friends had come in to support us ...so somebody asked what had caused my brother's death and my sister said: 'Oh he had AIDS'. There was shock in the room and my uncle looked at her like: 'Oh God!'. This is because we were not expecting her to just talk like that ...Strangely, all those people present kind of knew what had killed him because the symptoms had been very clear. ... But I guess it's always better not to mention these things because they are shameful even when one is dead. The shame is even seen to affect the family and friends as though they are not good people... Again there is the widow he left behind whom we needed to shield from the shame. ... (Gaudencia, Lecturer, Weruini).

AIDS hit my family 10 years ago through my in-laws. ... It was very traumatic because it was the worst time to have it, it was totally stigmatising. People didn't understand it and thought of all the worst things. What was actually very traumatising was that it was happening in a Christian family. My father-in-law was a church leader and when such things happen people are so quick to point fingers. This has been a big family secret as my husband did not even tell me that it was AIDS until the parents were long gone ... I didn't even tell my own family about it ... Years later, I learnt that my sister too was infected. I was shocked but she is very positive about her status... you are the first person I am telling this outside our family ...telling people only gives them a chance to point fingers.... (Mrs Munyi, Lecturer, Weruini).

All the above extracts indicate that the shame associated with sex had contributed to the denial and silence that was apparent in the two universities. As long as silence continues, it may not be easy for institutions like universities to develop practices which pay attention to the effects of this epidemic on the staff, hence taking into consideration gender aspects that this study has highlighted (see also Chapter Eight). The women I interviewed mentioned social status and Christianity as causes for the shame and stigma when a family member got infected (see also Chapters One and Seven).

The Discourse of Gendered Shame and Stigma

This shame that is linked to sex has some gender implications. As the findings of this study suggest, it makes women, especially educated ones, even more silenced and ashamed to bring to the fore their experiences with AIDS. Whereas both men and women in the modern African context may find it difficult to talk about sex because of the shame associated with it, colonialism and missionaries made it even more shameful for women(Arnfred, 2004; Baylies, 2000; Campbell, 2003; Campbell et al., 2006; Hunter, 2003; Machera, 2004). Hunter (2003), for example, notes that missionaries "had always viewed African women as the repository of the evil and dark side of African culture because of natural attitudes towards sexuality" (p. 171). The colonial doctors on the other hand were not interested in African women. They concentrated their efforts on determining male fitness for work (Hunter, 2003). It was only after the Second World War that these doctors, "charged with a new responsibility to maintain large and productive forces in the colonies became concerned that women's birth and fertility rates had declined" (Hunter, 2003: 171).

The colonial hangover may have contributed to how women have been viewed with regard to HIV and AIDS and indeed how the women themselves view the situation as I discussed earlier in the present chapter. The following are two examples of what the women in this study said regarding stigma and shame:

> The reasons why people won't come out publicly to admit their HIV status is due to fear. One will ask: 'how will people take me? What will they think of me? How will they treat me?' And that stigma makes one decide to live with the disease quietly – I can tell you this is what is killing people (Mrs Mwithaga, Librarian, HG).

> Recently a colleague mentioned a staff member who was infected and the person was referred to my office...I waited but she never showed up ...I think she was ashamed to face me, especially if she was a born again Christian and may have feared what I would think ...we are professionals but people still fear...I later learnt that her employment was terminated... (Ms Kibet, Counsellor, HG).

As the above two examples suggest, the linking of AIDS with sex and immorality continues to perpetuate stigma and shame leading to silence. This silence makes it difficult for institutions to plan for affected or infected members of staff. Equally, institutions do not want to face the reality that their staff members could have been 'immoral' (like the case of Holy Ghost discussed in Chapter Eight).

The stigma and shame in universities is not unique to Holy Ghost and Weruini as noted by Lindow (2006) in the case of the University of Zambia:

> I've asked lecturers to break the stigma' says Mr. Tembo. 'If two or three lecturers can come out in the open, it will make the students realise that there is no need to hide. They all told me to my face: you must be joking. I can't be open. How will I teach my students if they know I am positive? (p. A69).

The stigma in the University of Zambia continues although they have one of the best AIDS treatment programmes amongst African universities (Lindow, 2006). My argument is that reducing AIDS-related stigma would probably help to achieve more sustainable AIDS initiatives, especially where women are concerned. This could be achieved if the discourse of sexuality was to change from

Sexuality, Silence and Stigma

immorality and blame and probably focus on issues of sexual rights and pleasure.

The Discourse of Blame

Other reasons why it has proved difficult for universities to rise up and face the truth about AIDS go back to the politics, which have been associated with this pandemic. From the 1980s when AIDS became a problem of concern globally, there has been some sort of a blame game and finger-pointing regarding its origins. The main discourse in the early days of the pandemic was that it originated from Africa (Hunter, 2003; Mbilinyi and Kaihula, 2000; Sabatier, 1988; Vliet, 1996). The myth then was that "if you are African, you are at risk...prostitutes are named directly, the implication is that large numbers of African women behave as if they were prostitutes!" (O'Sullivan, 1996: 87).

In Chapter One, I have noted that there are still contradictions in the way the global community views HIV and AIDS. Such contradictions extend to the way the HIV and AIDS problem has continued to be handled at the grassroots where people are dying in large numbers. Even though it has been globally acknowledged that the AIDS-related stigma is becoming a bigger epidemic than the disease itself, there seems to be very little change of attitude. In addition to the sexual stigma and shame discussed earlier in this chapter, the situation of AIDS has worsened since it has spread most dramatically in sub-Saharan Africa compared to the rest of the world. On this Hunter (2003) has noted:

> Early research into AIDS in Africa helped perpetuate the notion that African sexuality is bizarre and uncontrolled by focusing on 'ethno-pornographic' details like dry sex and intercourse with virgins and children. African commentators reversed the tables and argued that AIDS is associated with the 'perverse' Western practice of homosexuality (p. 175).

As a result of all this confusion and pointing of fingers, Hunter (2003) further notes:

> In the end, serious diseases go undetected and unreported because of shame, and sexuality gets channelled into violent and exploitative expression, driven underground by shame. The same prejudices and fear that hindered responses to STDs throughout history continue to hamper our responses to HIV and AIDS in the world. The result? Unimpeded, frightening growth of the disease in country after country and the build-up of an enormous disease reservoir that mocks our prudishness and threatens our survival (p. 175).

My interpretation of the AIDS discourse of blame is that it only helps to entrench and conceal the heterosexist and patriarchal identities and relationships that lead to the devastating effects that HIV and AIDS continues to have among women. I find McFadden's (2003) argument about this discourse appropriate when she notes:

> My contention is that only by stepping back from the noise and clamour surrounding HIV and AIDS as a disease can we reclaim our agency and begin to move beyond the horrifying places to which sexual domination has driven many women (p. 51).

From McFadden's contention above I now move to the next section to show how the blame game has continued to fuel AIDS-related stigma in the two universities under study, leading to a situation of 'non-action', as the preceding chapters have shown.

AIDS-Related Stigma and Silence in the Two Universities

The AIDS discourses discussed in the previous sections were manifested in the two universities leading to secrecy, denial, fear of stigmatisation and discrimination of those infected or affected (Kelly, 2001). The following sections provide examples of how this was happening.

Holy Ghost University

The two universities lacked a systematic response to the impact that AIDS was having on their staff (see Chapter Eight). Holy Ghost was worse in fuelling stigma under the guise of Christianity. In this section, I look at ways in which this was done using responses given by the interviewees:

> The problem with HG is that nobody encourages you to talk about some of these experiences I have shared with you. That is why I was saying that if we are ever to help ourselves, then our top managers should know it is time they started talking informally around these things so that we can be free to open up to them. If the university is only for academic business only, without bringing in any of our personal problems, then we shall only bottle them up and we will die of even stress and loneliness – not just of AIDS. … I think, in a Christian college, we have a bigger problem because of the thinking that we cannot be affected by such a problem because we are Christians…Yet even staff are not any different even though they may all claim they are born-again (Ms. Karabo, Lecturer, Holy Ghost).

In the above quotation, Ms Karabo observes that the silence and shame associated with HIV and AIDS amongst Holy Ghost staff is linked to sex and immorality. She supports my argument in this chapter, that linking sexuality to immorality offers little help to AIDS prevention strategies. This is because it silences certain groups of people (especially educated Christian women) who do not want to be associated with bad behaviour.

A study of two Australian universities (Currie et al., 2002) also showed that when universities focus only on business issues, pressures on staff tends to increase and exhaustion becomes more widespread. As a result, many staff may choose not to advance their careers, and just stay where they are.

The above mentioned study, though not related to HIV and AIDS as in my case, suggests that women's careers tend to suffer more when universities fail to consider personal and private lives of their employees. In the case of Holy Ghost University that Ms

Karabo was referring to, instead of remaining silent about HIV and AIDS, the university needs to have an agenda that cares for its employees, more so women. Dr. Kivuu confirmed Ms Karabo's concerns when he noted:

> We don't employ people if they test HIV positive...Well it's not discrimination or stigma – the point we are trying to make is that if you are a person who has Christian values, then you don't hope to get that kind of illness. As a private university, we are saying that the Christian values have to be kept. Consideration on who we take is based on the person's commitment to Christ...This is what we are here for and we should be able to impact on the society and the Church. What kind of impact would our staff make if they are coming with that kind of testimony – where they have been infected by a disease that comes with immorality – surely we have nothing to do with such people (Dr Kivuu, ACU Director, HG).

Such a position by management, as articulated by Dr Kivuu, could make women's private challenges to continue being unrecognised.

As I noted in Chapter Eight, the only woman manager I interviewed presented a different perspective from Dr. Kivuu's. Unfortunately Dr. Kivuu was the ACU director and the one charged with the responsibility of steering AIDS work in Holy Ghost. Mrs Mwala saw the need for management to be accessible to all staff so that they could talk about their problems without fear of discrimination:

> I think we need to change the attitude so that we do not relate AIDS with sin. That is the problem and actually one who fears God and is faithful to Him can become a victim not because the person has sinned. For example, there are people here who are born-again but their spouses are not born-again so they can as well fall victims. You can also be born-again and your husband is born-again and through blood transfusion, you get it. So actually what we need to do is change our attitude towards it (Mrs Mwala, Deputy HRM, HG).

Mrs Mwala's ideas are unlikely to influence policy and practices in Holy Ghost because she holds a more junior position compared to Dr. Kivuu's. Given the patriarchal structures in the university (discussed in Chapters Six and Eight) she is unlikely to rise beyond her current position. Even if she were to become the human resource manager, she is unlikely to influence the large number of men in top leadership.

According to Barnett and Whiteside (2002), HIV and AIDS mixes sex, death and fear in ways that suit the prejudices and agendas of those controlling the narrative at any particular time or place. In a Christian environment like that of Holy Ghost, moralising this disease has caused fear amongst the infected because they may be sacked. The role of the church in increasing AIDS stigma is highlighted by Campbell et al. (2006) when they note:

> The church teaches that sex should be conducted within a faithful marriage and that sex outside marriage is a sin. The HIV/AIDS epidemic highlights how many unmarried people are sexually active and it also highlights the way in which many people ignore the church's teachings. This shows that the church has lost some of its moral authority and power. One of the strategies that some representatives of the churches use to try and get back this lost moral authority, is to say that people with HIV/AIDS are guilty of sin and immorality and their behaviour may even lead to the end of the world (p. 135).

The argument in the above quotation reflects the situation in Holy Ghost. Even though Holy Ghost management were aware that their community was not adhering to the church teaching as far as sex was concerned, they continued to behave as though the problem did not exist there. In order to maintain their authority as a 'moral' institution, they resorted to getting rid of those infected, thus increasing silence and stigma.

Weruini University

In Weruini, unlike Holy Ghost, the silence and stigma was not directly linked to anything the university was doing. But rather, it was linked to what the university was not doing. Relating to how stigma was affecting staff in Weruini, Dr. Oduor, the ACU director, gave one example:

> One very senior person here came and whispered to me that he was HIV-positive. His worry was that his wife would know about his status. He had just been tested the previous week and his problem was how to disclose it to his wife and children. I don't know whether he eventually did tell them but I advised him to because at the end of the day chances were the wife was also positive... Our biggest challenge is stigma amongst our staff members. There are still very many who cannot come and tell us what their problems are.

Given the prevailing AIDS discourses in the universities discussed in this study so far, it can be implied that stigma presents a challenge that requires some intervention. Lindow (2006) raises similar sentiments when he notes the following about the University of Zambia: "the stigma of AIDS has thwarted the university's best efforts" (p. A68).

Openness about sexuality is needed if AIDS is going to be successfully tackled inside and outside universities, as noted by some of the women:

> If there was openness, even the ARVs could be in the health unit and they would be cheaper. Our culture has a lot to do with whispering... the silence in the university is a reflection of the society ... may be if we had been open as a society and more supportive, my brothers wouldn't have died so soon (Prof Atieno, Senior Lecturer, Weruini).

> Although the ACU has HIV testing days, few staff members ever turn up... It is also very difficult because I don't think staff members are enthusiastic about it...people are afraid that others might know their status... my guess is that we have many people infected and they fear to confirm the truth (Dr Atoti, Senior Lecturer, Weruini).

> I must confess that the silence has continued to make the stigma worse. I think it has hit students, academic staff, the support staff and us all. I may not be able to give you the figures 'off-head' but as I said earlier, this does not need a doctor to tell us so and so is sick, you see

the trend... people are sick, yet they cannot say what is ailing them... and as you can imagine, it's because people are ashamed of being seen as immoral (Prof Nyaboke, Weruini).

Weruini University also faces the problem of silence and denial, especially amongst senior staff even if it is said to be one of those universities that has made satisfactory responses to the AIDS crisis. From the quotations above, and the discussion in the entire chapter and the preceding chapters, it is clear that much more needs to be done to address the multiple silences in universities which AIDS has helped to illuminate (see the following chapter for a summary of the silences that emerged in this study).

One of the women in my study (Dr. Nkirote) talked of her concerns about the silence and shame associated with sex. She felt that as an academic woman she had a role to play to change the sex-related discourse. She was of the opinion that it would be best to work with young people using what she referred to as initiation schools (as I have noted earlier in the present chapter). These schools would be used as a replacement to the traditional initiation practices that I have discussed elsewhere in this chapter. Together with her colleagues, they had started a training programme for teenage boys and girls:

We have a group of 15 women academics calling ourselves the 'HIV prevention and rehabilitation project of Kenya'. It is aimed at preparing our teenagers aged between 13 and 19 years. We give this group guidance and counselling for one week every year. Last year, we had a group of 39 residents for one whole week. We handle many topics including sexuality. It's a better way of transition from childhood to adulthood than FGM. We also feel that this is one way we can help to break the silence surrounding sexuality, which increases the stigma of HIV and AIDS and also its spread (Dr Nkirote, Senior Lecturer, Weruini).

The aim of the above mentioned training programme is to create spaces where young people could talk about their sexuality and other challenges that accompany the transition from childhood to adulthood. Dr. Nkirote believed that their school was playing a positive role of breaking the silence on sexuality especially among

Christians, as she and her colleagues were all born-again Christians. Although I cannot tell the impact this kind of programme was having on young people's attitudes, it is one indication of attempts being made to be more open about sexuality.

Summary and Conclusion

From the issues that I have raised in the present chapter, I see a need to investigate sexuality beyond the Christian, colonial, patriarchal and finger-pointing approaches. This may not be an easy task and it requires a multi-sectored approach involving key organisations like churches, communities and educational institutions. Universities, supposedly being citadels of knowledge, have a moral responsibility to lead by example in changing the AIDS discourses within them.

From the preceding chapters, it appears as though the two universities that I studied have not done much to provide this kind of leadership to the rest of the country. The findings suggest that the two were perpetuating stigma by continuing to 'moralise' the disease and staying silent about the extent to which their own staff are affected. As Kelly (2004b) observes, there has been little realisation amongst members of African universities that they need to be in the forefront of the fight against this epidemic. However, efforts like those of Dr. Nkirote can be a good beginning, and it would even be better if they have no religious and moral undertones in such a way as to defeat the very purpose of our struggle against HIV and AIDS.

As Kenya, and indeed the whole of Africa, battles with the immense challenges that the rise of HIV and AIDS crisis presents, universities need to take a deliberate step away from debate and donor politics (much of which employ discourses that force us back to racial and gender stereotypes). Through research, the African university community needs to uncover the underlying sexuality crisis presently faced by our continent (Phaswana-Mafuya, 2005).

=10

Summary, Conclusion and Suggestions for Good Practice

Introduction

The present study has sought to explore the situation in two Kenyan universities where it seemed as if AIDS and gender issues, especially as they affect senior women staff, have not received much attention. The study utilised a feminist perspective, feminist methodology and qualitative methods of data collection. The methods used included conversational and focused interviews, AIDS policy analysis and field notes. A total of twenty senior women academics and senior administrators as well as four men and one woman representing senior management of the two universities were interviewed.

Drawing on women's experiences with HIV and AIDS as a reflexive device, my study has sought to demonstrate the embedded male structures in academia that hinder gender equality. I have used feminist concepts such as patriarchy, silence, discourse, 'personal as political' and care. I used these concepts to analyse the experiences of women (as professionals) who were affected by HIV and AIDS in order to answer my research questions.

In the data chapters (Six to Nine) I have tried to address four of my research questions. However, the difficult task that I face as I come to the end of this book is to try and show how the issues raised so far can be applied in Kenyan universities that are currently grappling with HIV and AIDS and the challenges it presents.

When I had completed writing the first draft of my research report (without this last chapter), I asked a senior male colleague (whom I call Dr. Gitee) in a private university in Kenya to read it and give me his feedback. Dr. Gitee is a senior manager in his university. He commented that my research had raised some interesting issues worth thinking about. However, he thought that it would be difficult for universities to be concerned about people's personal lives. Employees, according to him, should sort out their personal matters without expecting the employer to be involved. The role of the employer was to make sure that staff had the facilities they need to do their work.

As a manager, Dr Gitee separated the personal from the professional. This separation is discussed in Chapters Six, Seven and Eight and has been shown to exist in other universities (Currie et al., 2002; Onsongo, 2005). I argue that this kind of separation tends to make men privileged and women disadvantaged in the academy. This is because, as my research suggests, the women have to contend with heavier burdens in their private and personal lives so that their professional lives are affected.

My experience with the present research has indicated that the issues that my study raises may be difficult to implement, a point also raised by one of the women in this study:

> What you are doing sounds good but I think it is very impractical. Right now the teaching and administrative workload has been increased...Your employer has employed you as a worker and doesn't want to know what is happening in your private life and that's why when people start dying of AIDS, it's a private issue...Whatever you do after work is your problem... Is the university supposed to give me less work so that I can cope as a single mother? Is that not my private business and I should make arrangements the way I deem fit? ... It is a noble study but a hard one to achieve. I wonder if anyone will take your recommendations seriously (Mrs Musoga, Lecturer, Weruini).

If I were to defend my propositions to Dr. Gitee and Mrs Musoga, I thought the best way would be to allow the women in my study to speak. For this reason I decided to address the last of my research questions in this last chapter, which was: What suggestions did the women have for improving practices in their universities to make them more accommodating to women's needs? Some of the women's suggestions about some of the steps that can be taken to improve women's situation in their universities arise in the thesis and I include others in the suggestions for good practice later in this chapter.

In order to make more comprehensive suggestions that could be applied to a wider university community, I suggest that more research is carried out to establish the extent to which the situation in these two institutions mirrors other Kenyan universities, and those in the African continent. My research, however, provides a useful illustration of the absence of gender issues in the two universities studied and probably all Kenyan universities (see below in this chapter). The comments from Dr. Gitee and Mrs Musoga are indeed instructive of the silences about the issues that my study has raised. Their comments also remind me of my personal experiences that prompted me to carry out this research (see Chapters One and Five), which I reflect on further in this chapter.

In this final chapter I will address the following areas:

* My reflection on the entire research process and a summary of the research findings
* The strengths and limitations of this study
* Some conclusions
* Suggestions for good practice
* Contributions of the study
* My suggestions for further research

A Summary of the Research Process and Some Key Findings

At the women's workshop where my research question was 'born', I talked about my experiences as one affected by HIV and AIDS. The women's reaction showed that I had "said something publicly that they wanted to hear said aloud" (Gold, 1995: 101). Many women who whispered to me after my session said that HIV and AIDS had affected them. None of them (like myself) were aware of any initiatives in their universities that were dealing with the issue. The 'whispers' and lack of any initiatives in the universities to deal with HIV and AIDS, especially its effects on women, prompted my interest in this study, in which I have argued that HIV and AIDS has introduced new challenges into workplaces. These challenges have remained unspoken, unseen and absent in policy and practice of universities (Kelly, 2001, 2003b). These challenges may be new, but they also present a heightened example of common gender imbalances.

The present study is a long story of women's experiences in two Kenyan universities. It starts with my own dissatisfactions as an academic woman in Kenya, not only because I was affected by HIV and AIDS, which felt isolating as no one else was talking about the epidemic, but I had also experienced other hostilities, for example sexual harassment, and I was denied funding for my PhD (see Chapter Five). Women's experiences, especially regarding the double roles they play, combining professional work with care-taking roles for their families, form the central argument in this thesis. My interests lay in the fact that these experiences appeared ignored and unrecognised in universities' general discourses.

In order to understand the women's experiences, I found it necessary to provide some background to the social, cultural, political, economic and religious contexts in Kenya. This background helped me to analyse and interpret the experiences that the women shared in the interviews that I present in the data chapters (Six to Nine).

To justify my use of women's experiences and my own as a valid way of generating knowledge, my research and writing have been guided by a feminist perspective. This perspective has helped me to understand the different ways that women are silenced. I have focused on neglected aspects of women's lives, especially with HIV and AIDS. In Chapter Five, I explain the concepts that helped me to analyse the themes that emerged from the interviews. Even though I call this study feminist, I realised that in order to access male and female respondents, and for my work to be taken seriously, it was necessary that I did not mention its feminist or gender nature to my interviewees. This was necessitated by the fact that the academic community in Kenya has not fully embraced feminism, a fact I encountered in the pilot study and was also noted by Onsongo (2005). I considered this as ethical and justified because through this kind of research, women's issues can be known and hopefully acted on (see Chapters Five and Six).

Ethical issues were central to this study for three reasons. First, ethical considerations make the feminist researcher accountable for the knowledge they may produce when "interrogating their own constitution as knowing subjects" (Ramazanoglu and Holland, 2002: 102). Feminist research is about fairness, respect and promoting the good of others, thus ethics become central. Secondly, this was a sensitive study because I was asking women to talk about private matters that brought painful memories. In addition, some of the issues discussed were family secrets. The university community was also seen to have stigmatised the issue of AIDS and in some cases discrimination of the infected was also noted, yet the management would not want the truth to be revealed in a research project (see Chapter Four). Thirdly, I was also aware of the power relations that existed between the research participants and myself, many of whom held more senior positions than I. It was for these reasons that I decided to write a reflective Chapter Four about the ethical challenges that I faced.

In Chapter Four I also reflect on the sampling decisions I made. This chapter fitted well with the theme of my thesis – of speaking and writing about the 'unseen and the unspoken'. I noticed that ethical challenges about sensitive topics had not received much attention, especially in the area of researching women in Kenyan universities.

Reflexivity was central to the entire project. That is the reason I became reflexive and included the chapter on the ethical challenges. My interviews were also reflexive; for example, in my interview with Mrs Mwala, I noticed that she was a little hesitant to talk about her university. However, this changed as our conversation progressed after I spoke to her about my own experiences with HIV and AIDS and the silences I had witnessed at my university (also a Christian one).

There were many similarities between Mrs Mwala and I, we were in the same age bracket and status in the university. This made our power relations more equal than those of some of the older and more senior people that I interviewed, as I discussed in Chapter Four.

On power relations in research, Ramazanoglu and Holland (2000) note that, "...despite the differences in feminist approaches to knowledge production, the identification of power relations in the research process is generally seen as necessary" (p. 118). Therefore, pointing out to Mrs Mwala that I too was familiar with the way a Christian university operates, and the silences therein, made her more comfortable.

The interviews made several women reflect about issues in their lives in the universities and their careers that they had taken for granted. Many of them made comments like: 'I had not thought about that, I hope these findings can be disseminated to the senior management'. Prof. Nyaboke, for example noted, "I have never given the issues we have talked about much thought, but I know they matter" (quoted in Chapter Eight). My research, in essence, has been a process of making explicit issues in women's lives that have remained unrecognised in workplaces. I have used HIV and AIDS as the example to show how women's experiences are invisible in two universities. However, I have explored other areas that are also important to women's careers and which also appear to be unrecognised in the universities. Chapter Six presents the status of women in the senior management of the two universities. The chapter also explores the factors that the findings of this study suggest have hindered the career progression of women compared to men.

The study is saturated with women's stories and that is what I intended it to be. Stories, especially related to terminal illness like HIV and AIDS, have been said to be one way of facilitating healing (Gichure, 2006). Chapter Seven focuses on stories of how the women were affected by HIV and AIDS. In this chapter, I argue that the 'personal is political'. I also argue that women's care-giving responsibilities can have a negative impact on their university careers. The women's stories show that even though university careers are very demanding, women still have more domestic responsibilities than do men. The division between the 'public' and the 'private' only makes it harder for them to cope with university careers, as suggested by other researchers (Barnes, 2005; Kjeldal, 2005; Onsongo, 2005; Smit, 2006).

The two universities under my study were found to provide little support to women, but the women were expected to support students especially on welfare matters. Studies by other researchers suggest that men do not usually provide as much student support as women, while students do not also seem to expect as much support from male lecturers as they do from women (Deem, 2003; Morley, 1999, 2003a; Probert, 2005).

The women's stories presented in Chapter Seven lead me to ask another question: Were the universities doing anything in response to the painful experiences narrated by the women? In Chapter Eight, I explore the impact of and responses to HIV and AIDS in the two universities. What emerges is a situation of 'see nothing, hear nothing, do nothing'. Patriarchy and power are used to understand the lack of attention to issues affecting women in the two universities. In Chapter Eight, I argue that if policies are framed within a typical male perspective, even though they may sound 'women-friendly', the actual implementation becomes gender blind, as seen in Weruini University AIDS policy.

The findings of this study suggest that patriarchy dominated the AIDS discourses that were operating not just in the universities, but also in Kenya and globally. Colonialism and Christianity were also seen to have introduced a culture that especially silenced women on matters of sex and sexuality. Chapter Nine explores the stigma and silences around sexuality in the Kenyan context. Some of the dominant AIDS discourses are also explored and linked to the situation in the two universities.

Overall, a feminist perspective has helped me throughout this thesis, to see the unseen, name the unnamed and to unearth silences that existed in different areas of women's lives and in the universities. I now provide a summary of the silences that this study uncovered.

- *Silences about what is known but not taken account of:* This kind of silence is described by Treichler and Warren (1998) as:

  The power of the powerful themselves. The ability to keep an area silent and virtually unexamined is an important, if not ultimate key to institutional power (p. 140).

  This is the silence that comes through the discussion in Chapter Eight where the two universities studied had chosen to remain silent about the effects of AIDS on their staff, although they were aware of its devastating effects. In Chapter Six, I also explored factors that were seen to hinder women's career advancement. Some of the women had learnt to accept the status quo, leading to silence from the women and management.

- *Silence about issues which people may feel restricted to talk about:* I see the discourse of AIDS in Kenya as 'impenetrable' for educated women in relation to their own experiences. This is due to the fact that sexuality (in general) is central to the discourse of AIDS. Yet women in this study appeared restricted to talk about or engage in the discourse. Christian values that are deeply entrenched in Kenyan society seem to restrict women from talking about sexuality and have also linked women's sexuality to shame and stigma. This silence is discussed in Chapter Nine.

- *Silence about not knowing issues:* There is silence about issues that people (in this case women) "do not know that there is a discourse other than the one in which they function already" (Gold, 2001: 22). This is where professional women see no unfairness in the ways society positions them. Because of this kind of silence, women do not challenge the status quo. They appear to make choices that may jeopardise their careers, as long as their lives (especially their families) remain intact. They have accepted that good women should do everything to support their husbands and families, while still trying their best to manage careers. Many of the women had chosen 'the work hard' option as the best way to manage within the family and university structures. Those who went against this rule met ridicule from both men and women. In

Chapter Six, I gave an example of how Dr. Wangare was ridiculed by her colleagues when she told them that she was leaving her children to study in the UK. This kind of silence has been noted in other studies (Kjeldal, 2005; Morley, 1999, 2003b; Probert, 2005).

- *Silence about issues that are seen to belong to the private sphere*: Women may choose not to speak in public about matters that they think belong to private spaces and hence should not be discussed in the workplace. This 'choice' (one that is socially constructed) to remain silent for the women covered by my study was different from the kind of silence described above and the kind noted by Treichler and Warren (1998):

> Silence because women choose not to speak. This notion has an implicit power in it, a notion of choice...that transforms the 'silencing of' into the 'silence of' and grants some degree of power to the silent (p. 140).

Treichler and Warren (1998) are talking about feminists who chose not to talk out in the early stages of the AIDS crisis. In the case of women in this study, the decision not to speak could be associated with lack of space where they could speak, or their sense of powerlessness. It can also be attributed to their socialisation; that private matters should remain private and need not be discussed in the workplace since they are not the concern of the employer. This silence comes through in Chapters Six, Seven and Eight.

- *Silence and fear induced by Christianity*: Certain prevailing perceptions of Christianity were seen in my study to contribute to fear and silence, especially among the women in Holy Ghost University. Christianity in general was found to have demonised the AIDS epidemic and silenced people for fear they could be perceived as 'bad' if they were associated with the disease. A similar situation is noted in South African universities (Francis and Francis, 2006). Because of the advent of Christianity and colonialism, traditional forums where matters related to sexuality used to be discussed were discouraged, especially among the 'modern', educated women. My interviewees felt that they lacked appropriate times and places where sexuality could be discussed and brought into the open.

- *Silence about HIV infection*: This is another form of silence that became evident from my interviews. Only one woman said that she had been tested for HIV a year before the interview. Another said she had once considered going for a HIV test, but she feared that a visit to a VCT could raise eyebrows among her colleagues and students, if they discovered or saw her going to one. Similar fear is noted amongst the senior staff in the University of Zambia (Lindow, 2006). None of the other 18 women mentioned anything about their own HIV status. I chose not to ask them about it since I feared that would silence them. It was my hope that this research would help some of these women to reflect on their own HIV status as they did on the status of others close to them. This would enable them, if they were infected, to access help in good time.

- *Silence about women's sexuality*: As has been seen in all the extracts that I have provided in Chapter Nine, which focused on sexuality, none of the women mentioned that they were aware of any lesbian tendencies amongst them. Homosexuality remains a taboo subject in Kenya and, although some men are known to be homosexuals, lesbianism is hardly acknowledged (Machera, 2004). Homosexuality is illegal in Kenya, but in recent years some articles have been published in the local newspapers about lives of men and women living in homosexual relationships. However, this is an area surrounded by even more stigma and silence. Even those who give interviews to the press do not disclose their true identities for fear of societal hatred and anger (Mutiswa, 2006). Additionally, Machera (2004) observes that in many African countries, homosexuality is suppressed as an alternative expression of sexuality through isolation and a conspiracy of silence. Social sanctions against single women are some of the ways used to maintain heterosexuality as Machera (2004) observes:

> For example, even if women remain single and couple with no one, they are ridiculed and ostracised ...men do not respect single women,

poor or rich, literate or illiterate. In fact, such women are easily labelled as rebels or prostitutes ...moreover if women love other women, they are seen as deviant or sexually pathological (p. 163-2).

Six of the women in my study said they were single. Four of them had never married, though they were well into their late thirties. Going by Machera's (2004) observations, such women may not talk about other forms of sexuality even if they could have been involved in them.

Besides the silence on other forms of sexuality, heterosexuality (especially within marriage) was another topic that was not discussed even with husbands. The married women in my study generally hoped that their husbands were faithful or that they used condoms whenever they chose to have sex outside marriage. Women's needs for sexual pleasure were also unspoken. The sexual needs of the single women were also unrecognised. These silences may contribute to the continuing spread of HIV because partners are rarely open about each other's sexual behaviour (Hunter, 2003; Khathide, 2003; McFadden, 2003; Wood, 2002).

The Strengths and Limitations of the Study

The main strength of this study is that it has given a group of university women what Barnes (2005) calls 'the microphone or air time' to talk about their multiple roles in the context of HIV and AIDS. It is the first study that I am aware of in Kenya that has used senior university women's experiences with HIV and AIDS as an example of how their personal and private issues tend to go unrecognised in the workplace.

Using a feminist approach is both a strength and a limitation. It is a strength because women are made central. I have documented aspects of their lives that would not be seen as crucial in non-gender aware type of social science research, a point noted by feminist researchers such as Appleby (1994), Leonard (2001), Mauthner (1998), and Stanley and Wise (1983). However, this focus on women only is a limitation, which, though justified (see Chapter Three), does not provide a complete gender picture. I risk being seen to be equating gender to women. It would have been interesting to find out how men are also affected by HIV and AIDS. Indeed it has been suggested that there is a need to work with men in order to combat HIV and AIDS and to challenge unequal power relations and stereotypes (Bujra and Baylies, 1995). Later in the present chapter, I suggest the need for a study that would also include men.

Another limitation of this study was the fact that it focused on only two universities out of a possible 19 in Kenya (at the time of the study). The criteria for the selection of the two institutions are provided in Chapter Three. On the issues of gender inequality, the situation in Weruini and Holy Ghost is likely to be reflected in other Kenyan universities as there has been some work in this area that has consistently suggested this to be so (Kamau, 2001; Kanake, 1995; Khasiani, 2000; Manya, 2000; Onsongo, 2000, 2005; Teferra and Altbach, 2004). It is for this reason that I make some generalised conclusions and suggestions for good practice in Kenyan universities as far as gender issues among university staff members are concerned.

However, since this was the first study to document senior university women's experiences, in particular with HIV and AIDS in Kenya, it is difficult to tell whether the situation in the two universities would be reflected in the others. I had initially thought of carrying out a survey of all Kenyan universities to establish the HIV and AIDS situation, but I changed my mind due to the limitations of time and financial resources. Because of this limitation, I address my suggestions about HIV and AIDS to Holy Ghost and Weruini. Nonetheless, I see this study as a good starting point for studies covering more universities.

While as the researcher I cannot predict as to how the text I have produced will be interpreted, I find it useful to reflect on possible readings of my research. I am especially concerned about the interpretations by senior university women in Kenya. By focusing attention on HIV and AIDS, I have selected one aspect of women's lives. While I started my interviews with much broader questions about women's lives and their careers, which I cover in Chapter Six, I have increasingly focused on their experiences with HIV and AIDS. I realise that this has the danger of producing a distorted picture of women's lives. I appreciate that HIV and AIDS is not likely to be what preoccupies these women's minds. Thus, there is a possibility that this research could be harmful to the participants, delving into sections of their 'private' lives where they appear vulnerable.

In public, these women are powerful and they may not want to be presented as powerless and vulnerable. That these women see themselves as powerful can be implied from the majority of them choosing to be called by their titles (Prof., Dr. Mrs). While in Chapters Three and Four, I discussed how I tried to avoid any harm to the women, the stories in Chapter Seven present them as vulnerable. I see this as a limitation while also a strength of the study in that the lack of recognition of the 'vulnerability' of such women has led to the invisibility of issues that matter to them, as I have argued throughout this book.

Some Conclusions

In this study, I have used the global problem of HIV and AIDS to show how issues that touch on the private lives of individuals, especially women, end up having a direct impact on their performance at the workplace. Looking at problems like AIDS, and other related social challenges as isolated issues, thus not including them in institutional practices, can cause a drawback to women's career performance. In order for women to manage a balance between their personal and professional roles and hence compete on an equal footing with men, gender sensitive policies, practices and culture are required in Kenyan universities.

Based on the data and discussion about the low numbers of women in senior academic and administrative positions on the two Kenyan universities, it can be concluded that women have less successful university careers than men (see Chapter Six). This is mainly "because of stereotypes, prejudices and hidden discrimination based on the idea that women should not be allowed to rise to the top of their academic careers" (Miroiu, 2003: 78).

The AIDS discourse in Weruini and Holy Ghost Universities need not be 'one-dimensional', focusing only on its dramatic spread and devastating impact on infected people or those viewed to be at risk of infection. Rather, the AIDS discourse requires an analysis of the inter-related factors. These include addressing gender issues and dismantling patriarchal structures found to be dominant in the two universities. It is also necessary to recognise that social challenges like AIDS, which fall in the private domain of people, require space and action in the public discourses that inform the formulation of policies and their implementation.

The study has also shown the importance of investigating sexuality beyond Christian, colonial and patriarchal discourses. I have argued that a suitable discourse that will reach out to the wider society to reduce AIDS-related stigma is required. African scholars need to take the lead to challenge Christian and colonial ideologies, which have blamed African cultures, poverty and backwardness for the increased HIV spread.

I find O'Sullivan's (1996) assertion appropriate that:

> Developing a feminist framework in which to situate AIDS necessitates talking about a lot more than AIDS. As feminists, we are uniquely prepared to intervene in our own and other people's panic and confusion (p. 90).

Women need to reject this culture of silence in order to enhance their self-esteem and participation in the leadership development of the institutions where they work and communities in which they live. Kenyan women need to form strong feminist movements through which they can voice their issues as noted by Machera (2004):

> I am enthusiastic that society, as a result of the feminist movement must envision new sexual paradigms to change the norms related to female sexuality. Such paradigms should enhance the female sexuality, including issues of sexual pleasure and well-being, thus promoting basic sexual freedoms (p. 168).

Suggestions for Good Practice

The present study is the first of its kind in Kenya to intersect gender, HIV and AIDS and higher education management. I therefore expect there will be many others like Dr. Gitee and Mrs Musoga (see the introduction to this chapter) who will wonder how my suggestions can be practically implemented, given that such issues have not been raised before. My study has made one important contribution – that of 'speaking the unspoken'. I therefore make my suggestions for good practice as a beginning for dialogue, that even the 'unseen' can begin to be 'seen'.

This study has provided some illustrations of the silences, absences and invisibilities of women's issues in two Kenyan universities. The literature that I have engaged with has shown that this study is yet another example of how women's experiences are ignored in workplaces leading to persisting gender inequalities. Given that this study is another illustration of an old problem, I believe that the suggestions I make here can be applied beyond the two universities studied.

My suggestions for good practice are made in two areas: women's careers in Kenyan universities, and HIV and AIDS and women in Holy Ghost and Weruini Universities.

Some Suggestions About Women's University Careers

The findings of my study seem to suggest that there is need for the support of women in the following ways:

- *Support of women's academic careers*: This study has suggested that a successful academic career in Kenyan universities comes at a big cost for women. Generally, women support the careers of their partners. They would rather sacrifice their own careers for the sake of their families. This gives men the freedom to concentrate on their professional development. The women this study focused on were found to be facing newer challenges due to HIV and AIDS. This situation can be rectified if universities raised the level of awareness in respect to obstacles facing women's careers, starting with young women at undergraduate level. Another suggestion raised by Miroiu (2003) that I find relevant to Kenya is "educating men to feel proud in regard to (sic) their academically successful partners; educating men to offer partnerships and support for the careers of their wives" (p. 82). It would also be helpful to women if university policies were to take into consideration women's domestic responsibilities, making them more visible and allowing for their existence in planning and programming (McKie et al., 2001). This would be transformative because men and women who wish to or who provide care can do so without worrying that they would jeopardise their career progression.

- *Support of women's research*: Kenyan universities need to commit more funds to research about the experiences of university women's issues. Such research would also bring into light the caring work that is predominantly done by women. Because such work is usually free or voluntary and mainly done by women, it is not usually regarded as vital duty. It is, therefore, not usually included in mainstream research. Ideally, the findings of such research would be disseminated in relevant forums where all stakeholders in the university sector can get a clear picture of the challenges facing women. For women's research to be part of the university research agenda, Kenyan universities could introduce autonomous gender studies departments or faculties. Makerere University in Uganda, for example, has made some progress towards gender equality since they started a women's studies department and a gender mainstreaming division, both of which support women's research (Nyanchwo, 2005).

- *Establish women's support groups*: Women can use support groups to advocate friendly policies in universities. Kenyan university women need not give up the struggle to improve their welfare. Working as a group works better than individually. We can learn a lesson from women in Wyn et al.'s (2000) study where women who had risen to top positions said that their efforts had not been in vain. After 20 years of fighting and asserting their positions, they had finally seen universities change into more comfortable places for women. Women committed to gender equality need to make commitments to leave their universities better places for women than they found them. An example is what Dr. Kaiga and her colleagues did in Weruini University where they succeeded in putting more lighting on campus thereby improving security for the university community, especially for female students and staff members who live on campus (see Chapter Six). Such groups could be formal or informal, large or small, as shared by one woman:

> At least everybody should have someone they can open up to without fear. Some problems that are very personal can best be shared in small groups. Here at HG, we have prayer groups. I am in one where three of us pray together, we can talk about anything, even about our partners at home, and even about our sex life there is nothing we cannot talk about. We are so open, we are not embarrassed and we are sure that no one else outside the three of us will get to know. We have been in this partnership for the last five years and I have never heard anything revealed to anyone outside the group. That shows we have a lot of confidence with each other and that is how we survive, ...I remember an incident when I had a crisis in the morning and my friend was in a meeting and I had to ask for her to be called and she came out and we talked and hugged and she told me, 'you have to be strong', and I was able to go to class. Had she not been there, I would not have been able to teach that day (Mrs Wakaba, Lecturer, HG).

In the present study, I have argued that the women whom I interviewed did not have spaces in the university where they could talk about private issues like sexuality. However, towards the end of the interview, Mrs Wakaba mentioned that she had some close friends with whom she could talk about anything. Given the unsupportive working environment that this study has shown to be existing in the two universities (see Chapter Eight), such women groups can be safe avenues through which women can find support. They can provide a starting point for changing university cultures to be more supportive to women (see Chapters Six and Eight). I suggest that Kenyan universities make a point of acknowledging and supporting such groups as they can provide places where women can get support on private and professional matters.

Research on the micro politics of workplaces has also shown that people who move up in their careers do so through networking, mentoring and sponsorship as Lorber (2000) notes:

> The way people move up in their careers is through networking (finding out about job opportunities through word of mouth...), mentoring (being coached through the informal norms of the workplace) and sponsorship (being helped to advance by a senior colleague) (p. 273).

In Kenyan universities where women are only in a minority, as suggested in this study and those of others, it becomes increasingly difficult for them to exploit available networks. Women therefore need to form their own networks and mentoring programmes in order to help each other to not only break the 'glass ceiling', but also to continuously challenge institutional cultures that keep them in the bottom ranks.

I make the above recommendation aware of the fact that if universities initiate such networks, then the networks may end up being as patriarchal as any other services that are already available. However, what I have in mind is a situation where women themselves would see the need to come together and form networks for advocacy and other activism. This would be similar to what Dr. Kaiga talked about (Chapter Six). But as Dr. Kaiga noted, their group 'died out' after the VC who had supported them left. Leadership from top ranks of the university is important for such individual initiatives to become well rooted. As I have argued in Chapter Six, this would require that more women willing to 'make a difference' rise to senior management positions in the university.

For this to happen, many of the hurdles women face to rise to seniority that this study and others have pointed out would need to be addressed. At the same time, the more informal and friendship groups mentioned by Mrs Wakaba (quoted earlier in this chapter) could become more formalised especially through the initiative of senior women who may have benefited from them in the first place. Such formalisation would make them accessible to younger women joining the institutions who may require support.

I hoped the interviews themselves would begin the sensitisation about gender issues with the women. I noted in my field dairy that many of the women reflected on how they could help to make life easier for themselves and other women in their institutions. This may have become the start of their feminist journeys. Both Dr. Wangare and Prof. Nyaboke held senior management positions (head of department and dean respectfully) and I believe that if they are given more support, they could help to set up such a resource centre that other women may find useful. Later in the present chapter, I explain how I intend to use the findings of this study to sensitise women staff in Kenyan universities to work together to make the environment more women-friendly, not just with regard to HIV and AIDS, but also with other challenges they face as women.

Some Suggestions for Good Practice on AIDS Responses

The following suggestions ensue from the findings of my study:

- *Establish staff resource centres*: It would be useful if Weruini and Holy Ghost Universities pursue a systematic agenda to support senior women who, as this study showed, were greatly affected by HIV and AIDS, but lacked avenues of sharing their experiences. It would help to set up resource centres, specifically for staff members, where they can seek support for personal issues like counselling, child care, divorce, retirement, retrenchment, further studies, health, sexual harassment, housing and related issues. These centres could be run by professionals as is the case in the private institutions where the women said they preferred to go for help instead of their own universities. They can be run at cost-sharing basis, as long as they are kept at the standards that senior professional women would find comfortable and suitable. The 'I Choose Life' (ICL) model for students that was found to be working well in both Weruini and Holy Ghost could be tried for staff as well.

The limitation of having such resource centres would be that they could easily become stigmatised like others already available. The 'ICL' model came across as a good one because it was student-friendly and showed no signs of being an area where HIV and AIDS would be an issue associated with any shame, but a place where all students could feel welcome. Such a model could be tried for staff. However, this initiative would need to go hand in hand with education about AIDS-related stigma, especially where senior women are concerned, to include members of staff who are currently not served by the available provisions.

- *Change rhetoric into action*: Weruini University in particular needs to move away from just rhetoric to action. Drawing up policies that are not followed by committed action is not useful. A clear understanding and theorising of issues that result into the implementation of new policies is required before the documents are written. Women need to be actively involved in strategising on such issues so that policy documents can be relevant to all (Bennet, 2005).

- *Mainstreaming AIDS work*: AIDS responses can be mainstreamed in Holy Ghost and Weruini programmes and activities (Kelly, 2004a). According to Kelly (2004a), mainstreaming means that HIV and AIDS concerns become routine, so that policies, programmes and practices of the institution are informed by and take full account of the relevant HIV issues. This would require that institutional environment and values should change to allow all persons (men and women) to operate freely and address people's needs without discrimination.

- *Make AIDS initiatives visible*: HIV and AIDS responses need to be clearly felt by everyone working and visiting Holy Ghost and Weruini. This kind of visibility was lacking in the two universities. Even the women working in the institutions were not aware of what was happening. The proposed visibility could include regular talks about AIDS in meetings, and informal occasions where all people can be involved. It could also include putting notices around the campus, using newsletter updates, and being part of the lived culture of the institutions (Kelly, 2004a). These can be effective ways of breaking the silence that has persisted in the universities as shown by this study.

One woman suggested this kind of an approach when she noted:

> I think we need to hear more and more about HIV and AIDS in Weruini. For example, we have started a corruption prevention campaign and it was being suggested the other day that the VC should address us on the issue of corruption so that the whole institution understands the commitment. We need a similar approach to this pandemic as it is worse than corruption, I think it's this issue of opening up. Again funds need to be committed to this worthwhile course (Prof Nyaboke, Dean Weruini).

Universities need to put in place meaningful efforts to eradicate all forms of HIV and AIDS denial, stigma and discrimination. Examples of services that the two universities can start offering could include arrangements for medical insurance for all diseases. In Weruini, for example, only professors had a medical insurance that covered all diseases including those caused by AIDS. In Holy Ghost, the medical insurance did not include HIV and AIDS related ailments. It would also help to have sick leave that is well coordinated at institutional level rather than individual heads of departments deciding to do so on ad hoc basis. Institutions also require a regular monitoring of staff known to be infected, and supplying ARVs to all who need them. Universities need to continuously train staff who deal with AIDS-related issues so that they are up to date with current developments regarding the pandemic.

- *Management to provide leadership in HIV and AIDS initiatives*: The women suggested that in order for private issues like AIDS to be spoken about, leadership was required. In Chapters One, Two and Nine, I pointed out that in Kenya, educated people prefer not to talk about HIV and AIDS in as far as it affects them. The disease is still viewed as one that affects the poor, the immoral, and generally those seen to be at 'risk,' such as prostitutes, bar attendants and long distance truck drivers (as I have been mentioning throughout in the present study). Due to this attitude, many of the educated people (especially women) who are either affected or infected become silenced because they do not want to be identified with a disease for 'others'. One woman suggested the need for more openness using Uganda as an example:

> Looking at what countries like Uganda have done, we need to be more open and realistic about this disease because, even as we remain silent, we are still dying. Even when people die, it is never stated what killed them and we are left to speculate. There should be incentives for people to go for testing. When senior persons like the VC go for testing, they should have the courage to talk about their results, whether positive or negative. They should use the opportunity to explain to all that the value of knowing outweighs that of not knowing. Even at a national level, the President should also lead by example. Why has he never revealed his own status? We need people in key positions to lead   the way so that people come out of that fear (Dr Wangare, Lecturer Weruini).

The issues that Dr. Wangare raised go beyond HIV and AIDS. Leadership is required in dealing with some of the unrecognised and unspoken issues that my study has raised. President Museveni's leadership role in the work of HIV and AIDS in Uganda has been quoted elsewhere by Barnett and Whiteside (2002) and Kelly (2003a). The research findings presented in this book have provided a beginning for this kind of talk. Senior management in Weruini and Holy Ghost could provide leadership by beginning to talk about things that matter to all, including gender issues. Senior women too can make a difference (see Chapter Six). They can make a choice to 'speak' and challenge social stereotypes. This can help them to experience a sense of growth (Goldberger et al., 1987). Similarly, Thiam (1986) poses challenging questions about what she refers to as African women's silences:

> Black women have been silent for too long. Are they now beginning to find their voices? Are they claiming the right to speak for themselves? Is it not a high time that they discovered their own voices, that even if they are unused to speaking for themselves, they now take the floor, if only to say that they exist...that they have a right to liberty, respect and dignity? (p. 11).

Thiam (1986) challenges African women to speak out for themselves. She acknowledges that women finding a voice in male dominated societies will not be easy. The men who have continued to enjoy the privileges of voice will not easily give them up, but women need to speak against patriarchal structures that continue to dominate them.

The women's voices presented in my study suggest that women do want to be heard, but they do not always feel 'safe' to speak, especially when they work in places structured to silence them. My research work, albeit focusing on only a small number of women, has given them a chance to express themselves about issues they would otherwise not discuss in the university setting. Their own voices have made clear what it means to live their lives both as professionals and as members of wider communities. They have also spoken about what they would like to see as more accommodating working environments.

I suggest that Kenyan universities provide leadership in breaking the multiple silences that the present study has highlighted since they have detrimental effects on women's careers. In addition to providing leadership in breaking the silence on AIDS, university scholars can use the pandemic as a means for Africans to voice a different and original view to the world, as they have suffered most from this pandemic.

I agree with Francis and Francis (2006) as they write about the AIDS situation in the University of Kwazulu Natal in South Africa:

> The university as a leading academic institution...has a moral and ethical responsibility to address the issues of HIV/AIDS prevention as well as raising awareness about it (p. 44).

While I have noted under the section on limitations to this study that my suggestions for good practice regarding HIV and AIDS will focus on Weruini and Holy Ghost, universities should provide leadership on important issues like HIV and AIDS. It is for this reason that I suggest that African universities provide some leadership in the work of HIV and AIDS. They need to be centres of excellence as far as best practices on prevention, care and treatment of people affected and infected by HIV and AIDS is concerned (CHE and UNESCO, 2004; Kelly, 2003b, 2004b; Owino, 2004; Phaswana-Mafuya, 2005).

Some Contributions of this Study

This study has made contributions in three areas: to me as a researcher, the interviewees, and university community in Kenya and Africa.

To me as the researcher

As I pointed out at the beginning of this book, my research questions were informed by my personal experiences as one affected by HIV and AIDS. This decision was informed by my ontological position that when people share their lived experiences, then private challenges, especially those facing women, can find space in public policy. I suggest that one of the ways in which public policies in universities can include women's experiences is through making women's voices heard in the public arena.

Listening to 20 women talk about their personal experiences on varied issues, especially with reference to HIV and AIDS, has made me more aware of myself in relation to the pandemic and other personal experiences that I had taken for granted. For example, I have sometimes felt sad to be away from my family while pursuing my PhD degree. Listening to the struggles of those women who were studying locally as they tried to juggle between reading and family commitments, made me to appreciate the chance I have had.

I have also come to appreciate that if enough awareness can be created among men about the need to support their wives' academic careers, then more married women can take time off to study away from home. That way, they can be assured of completing their studies in good time. In addition, the struggles academic women undergo while studying locally can be communicated to university managements, thus opening possibilities for affirmative action when giving scholarships to study abroad. Such scholarships need also to consider family packages, especially where women with young families are involved.

In addition, I have come to understand women's private challenges in ways that I had not done before. This research gives me a voice to advocate changes in universities that would help reduce hurdles that face women in the struggle to advance themselves. From this study, I can respond to Dr. Gitee (mentioned earlier in the chapter) with more confidence, since research evidence tends to be trusted.

If one day I become a senior policy maker either in the university sector or elsewhere, I would make sure that I make a difference for women. The present study has taken me through a reflection that I would not have got from any other tool. I come out of it a transformed woman. For this I am very grateful to the women (see my acknowledgements) who facilitated the granting of the scholarship that has made this whole journey possible.

To the Interviewees

The study also provided the women interviewees with a platform to talk and reflect on issues many of them had not had a chance to discuss. The study itself provided an opportunity to break the different silences that I have highlighted throughout this study. This was shown by the fact that many of them said that some of the issues they discussed with me had not been shared with anyone else before. This included their opening up about the effects of HIV and AIDS on their families and other personal issues. For example, one woman said I was the first person amongst her professional colleagues that she had told about her separation from her husband. Another interviewee, who talked about frustrations she had gone through while trying to get a PhD scholarship, said that this was the first time she had had an opportunity to talk about the experience. She asked me to give her the transcribed text as that was the only record of what she believed was an important part of her professional life and she thought that if she were ever to write her autobiography, then her interview with me, as recorded in this book, would be useful.

To the University Community in Kenya and Africa

Beyond the women I interviewed, and I, the present study makes an important contribution to the university community in Africa in general, and in Kenya in particular, in terms of highlighting issues affecting women in academia. Unearthing the different silences provides a beginning for dialogue that university women can use to empower themselves. Women can begin to make their voices heard even on areas they may not have considered possible, such as sexuality.

So far, I have managed to present the findings of this study in two conferences. I also presented the findings at the launch of an AIDS Control Unit in one of the private universities in Kenya. The feedback I received from senior management during this function was an indication that the university could begin to act differently (the Vice Chancellor, a woman, was very interested in the findings of this study).

An article based on this study has been published in the Women's Studies International Forum (Kamau, 2006). I intend to continue publishing the findings of my present research in academic journals and public media like the Kenyan daily newspapers. I believe that the dissemination of the findings of this study will prompt debates about the issues raised and probably be a beginning for positive change.

I intend to discuss the findings of this study with UNESCO and CHE (two very senior women in these two organisations are aware of this research and are keen to know the findings). These two institutions are already working with Kenyan institutions of higher learning on issues of HIV and AIDS. I hope we can work together in workshops on dissemination of such knowledge. We could begin with Weruini and Holy Ghost and probably move to other institutions. This might be one of the ways in which we could influence the policies that are yet to be written, as well as revise those written and influence programming where work has already began like in the case of Weruini.

Some Suggestions for Further Research

The following are areas where I think more research is needed to enrich the findings of this study and to cover areas that this study left out:

- A wider and generalisable study, sampling women from all the universities in Kenya and other African countries would help to give a more representative picture of women's experiences with HIV and AIDS and other related issues especially falling in the private domain.

- A similar study comparing men and women's experiences would also provide data on how men are affected by HIV and AIDS. It would also look at how different or similar their experiences are with those of women.

- Action research is needed, where some of the suggestions made in this study can be tested and tried in one institution. And with regular evaluation, it might reveal what works and what does not work in order to design a manual for better practice that can be used in other workplaces.

- There is need for a feminist research that would investigate African sexuality beyond Christian, colonial and patriarchal discourses. Such a research could also look into different types of sexualities and issues of sexual rights. The findings of such a study could help in changing the sexuality discourse, and contribute towards reducing AIDS-related stigma.

Appendices

Appendix 1

Kenyan Universities and their Status as at 2012

Name of University	Category and Status	Date Awarded Status	Religious Affiliation
1. University of Nairobi	Public, fully accredited	1970	None
2. Moi University	Public, fully accredited	1984	None
3. Kenyatta University	Public, fully accredited	1985	None
4. Egerton University	Public, fully accredited	1987	None
5. Jomo Kenyatta University of Agriculture and Technology (JKUAT)	Public, fully accredited	1994	None
6. Maseno University	Public, fully accredited	2001	None
7. Masinde Muliro University of Science and Technology (MMUST)	Public, fully accredited	2007	None
8. The University of Eastern Africa, Baraton	Private, fully accredited	1991	SDA
9. Daystar University	Private, fully accredited	1994	Protestant churches
10. Scott Theological College	Private, fully accredited	1997	AIC
11. United States International University (USIU)	Private, fully accredited	1999	None
12. St. Paul's University	Private, fully accredited	2007	Protestant churches
13. Pan Africa Christian University	Private, fully accredited	2008	Protestant churches
14. Kenya Highlands Evangelical University	Private, fully accredited	2011	Protestant churches
15. African International University	Private, fully accredited	2011	Protestant churches

16. The Catholic University of Eastern Africa (CUEA)	Private, fully accredited	1992	Catholic
17. Africa Nazarene University	Private, fully accredited	2002	Nazarene Church
18. Kenya Methodist University	Private, fully accredited	2006	Methodist Church
19. Strathmore University	Private, fully accredited	2008	Catholic
20. Kabarak University	Private, fully accredited	2008	AIC
21. Mt. Kenya University	Private, fully accredited	2011	None
22. Kiriri Women's University of Science and Technology	Letter of Interim Authority	2002	None
23. Aga Khan University	Letter of Interim Authority	2002	Ismaili
24. Gretsa University	Letter of Interim Authority	2006	None
25. Great Lakes University of Kisumu	Letter of Interim Authority	2006	ACK
26. KCA University	Letter of Interim Authority	2007	None
27. Presbyterian University of East Africa	Letter of Interim Authority	2007	PCEA
28. Adventist University of Africa	Letter of Interim Authority	2008	SDA
29. Inoorero University	Letter of Interim Authority	2009	None
30. The East African University	Letter of Interim Authority	2010	None
31. GENCO University	Letter of Interim Authority	2011	None
32. Management University of Africa	Letter of Interim Authority	2011	None
33. Nairobi International School of Theology (NIST)	Registered	1989	Protestant churches
34. East Africa School of Theology (EAST)	Registered	1989	Protestant churches

Source: *Accreditation and Quality Assurance Report July 2006 to June 2012*, Commission for High Education (2012)

Appendix 2

Researching a Sensitive Topic – Some Field Guidelines

Based on my readings and experience from my pilot study, the following were my field guidelines:

- Must have a **diary** with me all the time and make notes on it as soon as I can find space to do so. This will especially be helpful for my observations.

- **Negotiating access** – What am I ready to give back? If asked I will promise to give a summarised report of the findings, and some guidelines on best practices for university based on the findings of the study.

- Being wary of **gatekeepers** – Experiences from the pilot taught me on the need to have more than one gatekeeper; the need to avoid over reliance on one or two persons.

- Being very careful about the selection of the **interview context** – and this will depend on the respondents, in the introduction and request letter of telephone conversation. I will ask them to decide the best place and most comfortable for them. If they allow me, I will also suggest venues.

- My **introduction** to the respondents: be careful on the amount of information given about the study; will be different for the women participants and the decision makers. Given the sensitivity of my topic touching on issues like gender and sexuality and in a sensitive context on such matters (university) it will be helpful that I attend seminars and conferences, continue writing on these topics in the newspaper so that potential respondents can understand my position. This has been shown by other researchers as a way of helping to reduce suspicion when dealing with a sensitive issue. In dealing with a sensitive topic and context, it is important that potential interviewees understand the researchers' values and ideals as this gives them the confidence to share experiences about their lives. I have experienced this with the kind of feedback I get from people who read my opinion articles in the newspaper. Some of those I interviewed kept referring to some of these articles and they felt they could trust me with their own experiences. I will attend seminars throughout the research period where I can present papers and also get to meet more potential respondents.

- **On consent** – I need to be aware that it is very difficult to have a fully informed consent especially for the interviews with women, it is not possible for a respondent or even a researcher to really be clear of what the consequences of talking about private matters can entail (Hollway and Jefferson, 2000). I will try my best to 'do no harm'; nevertheless I need to be aware that it may be difficult to predict whether talking about some intimate and emotional matters will do no harm not just for my participants, but also for myself. The only solution I can offer is to provide a list of agencies where further help can be assessed. This will apply also to myself. I will require some debriefs if and when I need them. I will ask some close friends to keep an eye on me and alert me if they notice that I am getting stressed out. I will also 'listen' to signs of stress.

- On **power relations** – I need to be constantly aware of the power relations between my research participants and myself. Some of the factors that will have an effect on this are positions of the interviewee in relation to me, the context of the interview, gender and age.

- On **disclosure** of sensitive issues by my participants and myself. I need to be aware of the need to keep assuring them that the information will be treated with outmost confidence and all details will be kept anonymous and where necessary, I will change some of the details (e.g., age, ethnicity, position at university, etc) as long as these changes do not affect the quality of the data.

- **Endings** – I will be very careful about ending the relationship with the interviewees. I will do a well summarised closer with 'thank you' messages, after every interview and send a 'thank you' note to each one of them. I will not refer to the interviewees if I meet these people after that unless of course they initiate a discussion in this.

- How will the findings be **disseminated**? In case this question is asked, I will say that it is first and foremost for my thesis. However, after the PhD I intend to publish articles in journals and hopefully write a book that can be accessed by those outside academia. If the two case universities request for a report of the research, I can give them a summary of the findings, recommendations and some guidelines for good practice after completion of my studies.

Appendix 3

Introduction letter to the Vice Chancellor of HG University

Nyokabi Kamau,
Box 48379,
Nairobi, Kenya

15th September 2004

Vice Chancellor,
Holy Ghost University

Dear Prof.,

RE: RESEARCH ON 'UNIVERSITY RESPONSES TO THE HIV AND AIDS EPIDEMIC' – REQUEST FOR AN INTERVIEW

I am a lecturer at the Catholic University of Eastern Africa, but currently a doctoral student at the University of London, Institute of Education. I am conducting a research on what universities have done in response to the HIV and AIDS epidemic in relation to staff members, the experiences learnt so far, challenges and what is seen as the best way forward. I am requesting you to share with me your experiences on this.

This will be done in the form of a short interview where I hope you will share your experiences and views on this very important issue. I am kindly requesting you to allow me to tape record the interview. The interview should last for about 30 minutes. Pseudonyms will be used for both the university and yourself and nowhere in my report will the real names be mentioned.

Kindly let me know the most convenient place and time when we can talk without being interrupted. I will follow up with a telephone call to your office to confirm when we can have this interview. In case you would like to contact me, my telephone contacts are 0722-329420 or 4440184 or e-mail nyokabikamau2@ yahoo.co.uk. Your time will be truly appreciated. Thanking you in advance

Yours truly,

Nyokabi Kamau

Appendix 4

Introduction Letter for the Focused Interview

I am a doctoral student at the University of London, Institute of Education. I am conducting a research on what your university has done in response to the HIV and AIDS epidemic in relation to staff members, the experiences learnt so far, challenges and what is seen as the best way forward. I am requesting you to share with me your experiences on this.

This will be done in the form of a short interview where you will share your experiences and views as a senior person in your university. I am kindly requesting you to allow me to tape record the interview. The interview should last about 30 minutes.

Kindly let me know the most convenient place where we can talk without being interrupted. My telephone contact is 0722-329420 or 4440184.

Thanking you in advance

Yours truly

Nyokabi Kamau

NB: This information was given on phone and in some cases face to face, only in two occasions did I send a letter.

Appendix 5

Introduction Information to the Women

My name is Nyokabi Kamau, a lecturer at the Catholic University of Eastern Africa. Currently, I am a doctoral student at the University of London, Institute of Education. I am conducting a research into university women's experiences with HIV and AIDS, and generally to find out if their personal and private experiences are taken into account when universities make policies and take action to deal with issues. I am requesting you to share with me your experiences on this.

This will be done in form of a fairly relaxed conversation, and am kindly requesting you to allow me to tape record the conversation to allow for accurate record of our conversation and indeed to also allow us to talk without interruption of note taking. The conversation should last about 45 minutes.

Kindly let me know the most convenient place where we can talk without being interrupted. I will follow up with a telephone call to your office to confirm a convenient time and place for the interview. In case you require any further clarifications, please contact me on 0722-329420 or 4440184 or e-mail – nyokabikamau2@yahoo.co.uk

Thanking you in advance

Yours truly

Nyokabi Kamau

NB: I used this letter as a guide to introducing myself to the women, either face to face or on telephone. I did not send a letter to any of the women participants – but I had prepared it just in case I was to need one.

Appendix 6

A Guide to the Conversational Interviews with Women Staff

Warming up – introducing myself, mentioning the objective of the study (which I would have already explained when booking the appointment but a reminder is good), explain that this should take between 45 minutes and 1 hour, setting up the tape and just making sure that everything is okay (is it a safe place to talk without fear that someone might interrupt). Might we need to change venue? Might we need to put off our mobiles? Do we need a cup of tea before or after?

Background data – age, ethnicity, marital status, children, position at university.

Introduce the issue of HIV and AIDS and find out in a conversational manner if she is affected and have a talk on how, and in which ways she has been involved in care, and how this affected her personal and public working life, we can talk about coping mechanisms applied depending on how the conversation progresses, issues of silence, blame, stigma related to AIDS may come up, I can probe about them if not coming out as we talk – the guiding question in this section will look like this:

- Please tell me if you are affected by HIV and AIDS and how

- Are you directly or indirectly involved in providing support to persons living with the HIV virus – now or in the past? Please tell me more about these experiences

- Who/what has been your main support as you go through all these caring experiences

I can then move the conversation into personal level – after we are both more comfortable talking about others.

Introduce issues of AIDS, sexuality and stigma

Talk about the challenges of bringing personal issues to the workplace. The guiding questions in this section were:

- Have you been able to talk about these experiences (mentioned above) with colleagues at the university?

- Or is there any support system you are aware of that staff can make use of when they have challenges in their private life?

- Is there a forum where you feel free to talk about sexuality issues in the campus with colleagues? Or have there been seminars where such issues have been discussed for staff members.

- How have issues of blame, stigma and silence as they affect staff members being dealt with?

- Do you think it is necessary for staff members to have a place in the university where their private challenges can be discussed?

- Do you feel your private/ personal challenges affect you career growth? In which ways?

After this I will move the conversation to issues of policy and how the woman views how her university has responded to the epidemic, views on the general university culture, whether gender issues are taken on board when taking policy decisions – taking the example of AIDS. I will explore suggestions on best practices that could be adopted by her university. Guiding questions in this section:

- What has your university done so far that caters for staff members experiences with HIV and AIDS (either as effected and/or infected)

- How effective?

- Any suggestions you may have on best practices – that also take women's experiences into account?

Summary and closure – I will summarise the interview so that the interviewee can get some feedback at this point. This can indeed create a chance to bring forth some information that may not have come out during the interview that may also be significant. After this I will courteously end the session and thank the woman for her time. A thank you note will follow this.

Appendix 7

Guide to Focused Interviews

Warming up, introducing myself and objectives of my study, allowing the interviewee to ask anything before we start, explain that this will take as short a time as possible –may be 30 minutes. Other background data to include, position of the respondent at the university, gender, and whether directly involved with AIDS work at the university.

The interview was guided by general topics with prompt and probing questions under some subheadings:

On impact of AIDS on staff in your university:

• What are your comments on the impact of the pandemic on your staff members – both as affected and infected?

University's action:

• What is the current policy?

• Any initiatives like training – what has been the response?

• Any support available for staff that is infected and/or affected? Any facilities; for example, insurance, arrangements for housing those who have had to take on extra family members due to HIV and AIDS, provisions for flexible working hours – for those known to be ill and/or taking care of sick relatives?

Silence, stigma, denial, discrimination with regard to staff:

• What has been done by your university to break the silence, reduce stigma for those affected to pave way for more openness on this problem?

• Are there any plans on this? So that more people can feel comfortable to share their experiences, educate others and indeed help with prevention and care for those infected?

Best practice:

• What have you heard is being done by other universities in Kenya or in the region that you would consider as a good example of how universities should be responding to the pandemic?

- What in your view would be the best practice that your university can adapt to wholly tackle the AIDS epidemic?

Ending and closing:

Summarise what I have learnt from the interview, allowing for any last comments. Thank him/her and end the session. This will then be followed by a thank you note.

NB: This was just a guide; the actual sequence depended on each situation.

Appendix 8

An Example of a Transcribed Conversational Interview

Interview held with Dr. Wangare held in her office at Weruini on 25th November 2004 from 11.30 a.m. – she suggested we move out of her office (she was the head of department) to another she shared with a colleague who was not in the campus on the day. We were not disturbed in the office but she answered her cell phone once.

Nyokabi: Thank you for this time and accepting to be interviewed. Tell me something about yourself, a bit of your background.

Wangare: I am a Kenyan woman. I was born in Nyeri District of Central Province. Am from a family of six, three girls and three boys. Am from an Islamic background; my father comes from a purely Islamic background and my mother comes from a Christian background so she became a Muslim by virtue of her marriage. The first few years, maybe until my early adolescence we lived in slums in Nyeri town. Later we moved out to the countryside into a more peri-urban farm-like setting. I went to primary in Nyeri where I sat my Kenya Certificate of Primary Education (CPE). I was one of the very unfortunate ones who thought that I was smart in primary school but come the exam I didn't attain marks to go to a good secondary school. So I went to a private school where I sat for the Kenya Junior Secondary Education (KJSE). That became a turning point in my life. My father said I had to move out and join a teachers training college due to our large family which he could no longer support. I was barely 16 years old. By the time I was 17 years, I was standing in front of a classroom teaching. I was given the responsibility of educating my brother, but I also continued studying for the form four exam. It is a very long story so I can just put the highlights.

In the school where I was teaching there was a teacher who thought I was too young to waste myself. She got an interest in me and she kept talking with me. She was my mother's age and I remember her telling me 'you know you are so young and you will be sitting here at break time listening to women's gossips, as they talk about their husbands, their children'. She told me that I could do a lot with my life and she is the one who made me do the form four and form six exams. She made sure I was registered for these exams. This woman played a very central part in shaping my future....

I was a Music teacher and the choir mistress, the music patron joined me so we used to work together and we registered for private exams until I qualified to come to Weruini University for a diploma in Music education and Kiswahili and from then on studying became my hobby. After my diploma, I did my BA here and I got my scholarship for this particular department because I wanted to do my Masters... I decided to take Education so I applied to this department in communication and technology and I was taken... (A long discussion on this, which I leave out)

After I completed the MA and continued working, I realised I needed to pursue a doctorate. I told my dean I needed a scholarship, if the department could support me. I learnt that there were forms for commonwealth scholarships for PhD, which is usually given to government institutions. On learning about their availability at the university, I asked my dean to give me. The dean told me he didn't have them, that he only had the photocopy he had pasted on his door...I went to the registrar academic who told me the forms were finished and he only had copies... So I went to the British Council and they gave me...I did not send the forms through the university as I feared the dean may not forward them so I just sent straight to Cambridge ...I was admitted at Cambridge but without funding ... I needed to raise the funds so I wrote to Cambridge and I was told that year they had already disbursed their funds... I went to Ratansi Educational Trust who gave me 1000 sterling pounds per year for three years. I went to Aga Khan, they gave me 5000 pounds per year so I had 6000 pounds, but I needed 14,000 per year. After a year Ratansi withdrew their funding as I had not yet claimed it and I was worried I could also lose the Aga Khan money .... So I continued searching and at some point it was coming to a dead end and one day I got a letter from Cambridge instructing me to report in a month's time as the Cambridge trust had decided to give me the balance, my dear it was unbelievable! ...I put my children in boarding schools and left without study leave, which I was denied as the university claimed that I had not gone through them to get the scholarship so they had nothing to do with it....

Nyokabi When did you come back?
Wangare: I came back in 2001 April. I stayed for four years because I spent the whole of 1998 up to Feb 1999 in Kenya doing fieldwork then I started data analysis and then I went back part of 99 and 2000. I was already a lecturer by the time I left so when I came back the university regulations you have to either have completed 50% of your PhD or have completed so when I came back I applied

for a senior lecturer position and I got last year so now is to wait for the next step which is associate professor.

Nyokabi: Ok thank you so much for that background - Let's move on to HIV/AIDS what is your personal experience with HIV /AIDS. Have you been affected by this pandemic and would you take me through your experience if any?

Wangare: About HIV/AIDS. When you hear that every family is affected, for me it's a reality. What I can say is that every family or community is affected. That is a reality because let us say somebody like my brother's wife died in 1997 when I was away and it was confirmed that it was AIDS that killed her. My brother has been confirmed as HIV positive, he is still alive and I think it has been so depressing for him because he has deserted his job. In fact he left his job before his wife died. I think they knew what was happening and he decided to leave his job, take his cooperative money, do some business, which they never did so now he says he is another child in the family. I think he hasn't reached the point where he has AIDS and because of the depression and having no job, whatever little he gets he drinks chang'aa (illicit brew) and we have a resolution in the family not to ever give him cash. What we do is we go and get for him the necessities... whatever, he just does a small bit and he never does the rest. He has children and one of them is in form four, she is doing her 'O' level right now the other one is in class 8 and the other one is in class six and they all stay with my mother plus now my brother so that's why he's saying he is the child in the family. So for us it is a reality. It is something that has confronted our family.

Nyokabi: Are you involved in any way directly like taking care of your nieces and nephews?

Wangare: The burden is on the whole family ..... My mother stays at home ploughing the field so the income has to come from us so that is what has been happening. We support my brother and we pay school fees, the feeding and so on. I have particularly been very involved in supporting the children, I travel home regularly to see them and I also make sure that my brother takes his medication. I also try to support my mother emotionally. The whole family has been very supportive.

Nyokabi: Where do you derive or what can you say has been your main support or strength as you undergo your personal challenges?

Wangare: What I can say is that when I look at my CV right from primary school, what strikes me is how many women have been my pillars in life. That is what strikes me very strongly and starting from my own mother and then moving on to my colleagues. The kind of friends that I have had, and I have found that the support for women is so straightforward because it's like it has no strings attached, they help you without underlying expectation and without me imagining, you know sometimes there are no expectations, but we always imagine why is this person helping me, what might he want after that? I just find that there are so many women in my life like when I was employed here as a graduate assistant one of the lecturers who used to teach with me I say she is my mentor even in terms of teaching in class and even becoming a mentor beyond that in terms of research because I worked with her as a research assistant for a very long time getting very little money but getting a wealth of experience. I recommended her to be my field supervisor when I came to Kenya for my research. She was one of my supervisors because I was also taking a historical perspective. She has really mentored me all through even now I was with her on Monday and I look at other people in terms of social life who have stood by me when things were really bad...I find in my life women have been very very supportive without actually expecting anything...

Nyokabi: Here in the university do you have a group of women who you can.....say you count on in difficult times...?

Wangare: In this university is a bit tricky because of its nature. It is so expansive, in this department, for example, we have always had very few women because we are teaching history of education and am not sure too many women like teaching this, we have comparative education dominated mainly by men although we have like now one woman with a PhD and generally the staff has had very few women like now we have 23 men and out of that we have not more than six women in the MA class. I can say I have a lot of support because in the history of this university, I am the first woman to head this department. It has been a male dominated department. Imagine it is the men who campaigned for me saying that they wanted a woman head of department. I was not particularly amused because I was asking, what is the motive? These were the same people who had been leaving the job to their male friends and now they wanted me. I didn't take it as very sincere. I was very suspicious and thought maybe they wanted to tie me down here. It was a big issue because I wasn't a senior lecturer and the minimum for one to head a department is to be a senior lecturer unless there is no other senior person. They requested the VC that I was the best qualified for the job and after a year, the VC renewed it. I am on my second and last year. I have never understood why they wanted me, but they have supported me. The men even used to tell me that things have changed because in the past they would never allow women to head the department. They have even told me that there were other women but they never allowed them to head the department.

Nyokabi: Tell me about the issue of HIV/AIDS in this university. You have your own personal experience, you have your work experience. What is happening in the university as far as HIV/AIDS is concerned?

Wangare: There are things going on about HIV/AIDS, voluntary counselling and testing and I know that a few months ago real testing was going on in this university, the international day for testing and even our vice chancellor was in the forefront. So there is quite a lot of awareness we have a continuing counselling and testing taking place at our health centre apart from the HIV/AIDS unit. What I might not say in confidence is whether we have an institutional HIV/AIDS policy, which should govern the activities of a university so that we institutionalise these activities.

Nyokabi: Are you aware of any change the university has gone through now that we have a pandemic, have things changed the way they are run to accommodate this kind of a pandemic?

Wangare: What am saying is am not really aware of an institutional policy of that kind apart from the activities that can be seen clearly as addressing the issue. What I mean is if for instance we take the education sector, I know in many countries we have the HIV/AIDS policy in the ministry of education that is going to govern any educational institution and it's a clear policy on how people are being treated in terms of hiring and firing and how to treat students if they are infected or affected. So I cannot say in confidence that there is such a document in this university. I also know that there is a compulsory unit for all undergraduate students for one semester to cater for HIV/AIDS. In our department we teach a topic on it. We also have courses being taught at the centre for complimentary medicine at diploma and certificate level.

Nyokabi: How have these activities touched on staff members and especially on senior staff?

Wangare: Not one that is particularly targeting staff the way students are targeted. Because I know either sometime in August or September as members of staff, management staff, we were invited to participate in a workshop, which was being spearheaded by the AIDS control unit. What I saw there was a kind of sharing, but I don't know whether we can say that is something that has gone and touched the critical aspect of our lives in terms of HIV/AIDS. We went and listened seminar and people shared what they do, but on a deeper/ critical level where people sit and start reflecting on how they are fitting in the bigger picture that has not come in.

Nyokabi: This brings us to the next issue how do you find this university in terms of giving people space to bring in their personal or private challenges?

Wangare: Am not aware of any because it's like this university has reached a point where people tend to operate kind of individually and I think it's something that has to do with an institutional culture. Staff can't come together and share and be able to be happy together. I don't think we really create such spaces and I want to give an example of this department, we have a tearoom and it is something that I really had to fight for because it was being abolished. I took up that issue and it even reached the VC's office. I remember telling the dean if that room is going to be abolished then the teachers are going to be using his office because it means we have nowhere else to meet. That means I'll be coming from my house to the class and back. I think that is something that is going systematically, removing common rooms where teachers can meet. So that you are an individual, you cannot share, you cannot strategise. There is no sharing because there was a fear of people getting together and those are the spaces where people now share and they know who and who has a problem and how we can respond to that. So for this I know we really had to fight, the dean had to go with us to the VC, when we went the secretary was saying 'no the VC is in a meeting' and the dean said 'we shall wait here and as we wait students are in class waiting for us to teach' and I remember the dean telling his seniors that they also take tea so why can't a department be given its space to take tea? So eventually the VC had to make an executive ruling. I don't see any deliberate effort to bring the staff together. Unless this will be introduced in our new strategy which am a member we are writing a new ten-year development plan and those are the issues that staff (because we've collected information from all departments) that's what the people are raising they don't have space.

Nyokabi: From your experience, reading and writing what would you recommend as practices that would be good to be taken up by university in a time like this when we have this pandemic that would help and motivate people?

Wangare: I am happy you talk of good practice because there is talk of best practice, which I wonder if best practice exists.. one thing when we talk of this best practice first of all I have a problem with these practises and am happy because I believe if you talk of good practices then we have something to look forward to. From going around firstly we should start by having a very clearly stated policy and am happy if you are going to talk to some of our top administrators. They can tell you because for me I could say we start with a policy. If it's there then I am not aware or its not being communicated to the department. So we start from there and we need for people to participate in this policy and include issues, which we can think are our needs, what we think are our challenges, and what we think as a university are our strengths in addressing this pandemic and then looking at those challenges and the needs we have we formulate a policy that is responsive to these needs. Then it will be necessary to communicate this policy to the whole university community. But one thing I wouldn't really recommend is for a few groups of people, a committee, being called to come and strategise the HIV/AIDS policy maybe some people who are not even touched by this.

I would wish that it be as participatory as possible because the wider view would make it more responsive. Looking at what countries like Uganda have done, we need to be more open and realistic about this disease because even as we remain silent, we are still dying. Even when people die it is never stated what has killed them, we are left to speculate. There should be incentives for people to go for testing and when senior persons like the VC go for testing, they should have the courage to talk about their results, whether positive or negative. He should use the opportunity to explain to all that the value of knowing outweighs not knowing. Even at national level, the president should also lead by example, why has he never said his own status? We need people in key positions to lead the way so that people come out of that fear.

Nyokabi: And with that actually I think I have come to end; I have finished unless you would like to ask me something. As we went through maybe something came to your mind. Would you like to ask me something?

Wangare: I am just wondering why you narrowed your research on HIV/AIDS especially looking at university staff...

Nyokabi. I have narrowed my research to HIV/AIDS, because of my personal experience, I have had issues it in my family like yourself, close family members dying and I became affected in different ways such that even my work was affected – so from my experience I became interested in the issue.

Wangare: You know we just talk about how people are dying at this rate but we don't think about ourselves.

Nyokabi: So that is how I came up with the research problem, I really do not know what I will write but I am hearing a lot of experiences.

Wangare: I think you will have a lot to write as it is a major issue in our country. My best wishes...

(At lunch I was able to share my own experiences especially looking for funding, leaving the children, nasty comments from people, support from women, lack of support from universities for women's progression, etc. We had a very good sharing session. She requested I give her the transcribed text, which I did once it was transcribed. She emailed and thanked me for it.)

Glossary

Affected by HIV/AIDS: This term is used in this thesis to refer to persons whose close relatives have been infected by HIV or have suffered from AIDS. Such persons' lives become directly influenced by HIV infection and its emotional, psychological and sociological ramifications (UNAIDS, 2004a).

AIDS stigma: AIDS-related stigma (or more simply AIDS stigma) refers to prejudice, discounting, discrediting and discrimination directed at people perceived to have AIDS or HIV, and the individuals, groups and communities with which they are associated. This stigma leads to feelings of shame for the infected and affected. It also causes denial and silence among the affected and infected people.

Gender equality: The term is used to reflect an equal sharing of opportunities, resources and power between women and men. It also refers to equal access to education, health, administrative and managerial positions, equal pay for equal work, and equal political representation. Gender inequalities are seen to contribute to the spread of HIV and AIDS and to ways in which men and women are affected.

Gender: The term is used to refer to culturally specific patterns of behaviour, which can either be actual or normative and are attached to the sexes. Gender is a socially constructed way of distinguishing between males and females. It is what we learn to be as male and female. Ramazanoglu and Holland's (2002) view of gender is adapted, that "feminist knowledge of gender should include practical social investigation of gendered lives, experiences, relationships and similarities" (p. 5).

Infected by HIV/AIDS: This is a term commonly used to refer to those who have had a blood test whose results indicate they carry the HIV virus, which is believed to cause AIDS. People with the virus are generally referred to as HIV–positive.

Pandemic/epidemic: The words are used interchangeably throughout this thesis to mean a disease that is prevalent in an entire country.

References

Acker, J., Barry, K., & Esseveld, J. (1991). Objectivity and Truth: Problems in Doing Feminist Research. In M. A. Fonow & J. A. Cook (Eds.), *Beyond Methodology, Feminist Research as Lived Research* (pp. 133-153). Indianapolis: Indiana University Press.

Acker, S. (1994). *Gendered Education*. Buckingham: Open University Press.

ACU & DFID. (2001). HIV / AIDS: *Towards a Strategy for Commonwealth Universities*. London: Association of Commonwealth Universities (ACU).

Adkins, L. (2002). Sexual Servicing and the Labour Market. In S. Jackson & S. Scott (Eds.), *Gender: A Sociological Reader* (pp. 197-202). London: Routledge.

Adler, S., Laney, J., & Packer, M. (1993). *Managing Women*. Buckingham: Open University Press.

Ahlberg, B. M. (1991). *Women, Sexuality and the Changing Social Order: The Impact of Government Policies on Reproductive Behaviour in Kenya*. Philadelphia: Gordon and Breach.

Aisenberg, N., & Harrington, M. (1988). *Women of Academe: Outsiders in the Sacred Grove*. Amherst: University of Massachusetts Press.

Alderson, P., & Morrow, V. (2004). *Ethics, Social Research and Consulting with Children and Young People, Sensitive, Taboo Topics* (Revised ed.). Ilford: Barnardo's.

Alsop, R., Fitzsimons, A., & Lemon, K. (2002). *Theorizing Gender*. Cambridge: Polity.

Anafri, J. K. (2000). *Universities and HIV/AIDS in Sub-Saharan Africa - A Case Study of the University of Ghana, Legon*. Accra: ADEA Working Group on Higher Education The World Bank, New York.

Anderson, P., & Williams, J. (2001). *Identity and Difference in Higher Education : 'Outsiders Within'*. Aldershot: Ashgate.

Ankrah, M., E. (1996a). AIDS, Socio-Economic Decline and Health: A Double Tragedy for the African Woman. In L. Sherr & C. Hankins, et al. (Eds.), *AIDS as a Gender Issue: Psychological Perspectives* (pp. 99 - 118). London: Taylor and Francis.

Ankrah, M., E. (1996b). Let Their Voices Be Heard: Empowering Women in The Fight Against AIDS. *AIDS Captions Family Health International, 2*.

Appleby, Y. (1994, March 28 -29). *Listening and Talking: Interactive Conversation as a Feminist Research Method in Studying Experiences.* Paper presented at the British Sociological Association (BSA): Sexualities in Social Context, Sheffield University.

Arnfred, S. (2004). 'African Sexuality'/Sexuality in Africa: Tales and Silences. In S. Arnfred (Ed.), *Re-thinking Sexualities in Africa* (pp. 59-78). Uppsala: The Nordic African Institute.

Association of Commonwealth Universities. (2006). Commonwealth Universities Yearbook: A Directory to the Universities of the Commonwealth and the Handbook of Their Association (80th ed.). London: Association of Commonwealth Universities.

Bagilhoe, B. (1994). Being Different is a Very Difficult Row to Hoe: Survival Strategies for Women Academics. In S. Davies (Ed.), *Changing the Subject: Women in Higher Education* (pp. 15-28). London: Taylor and Francis.

Bahemuka, J. M., & Van der Vynckt, S. (2001). Empowering Women in The Community: The University's Role. In M.-L. Kearney (Ed.), *Women, Power and the Academy: From Rhetoric to Reality* (pp. 71-76). Paris: UNESCO.

Barnes, T. (2005, June). *Politics of the Mind and Body: Gender and Institutional Culture in African Universities.* Paper presented at the The African University of the 21st Century - SAARDHE, University of Western Cape.

Barnett, T., & Whiteside, A. (2002). *AIDS in the Twenty First Century: Disease and Globalisation*. Houndmills: Palgrave Macmillan.

Bassey, M. (1999). *Case Study Research in Educational Settings*. Buckingham: Open University Press.

Baylies, C. (2000). Perspectives on Gender and AIDS in Africa. In C. Baylies & J. Bujra (Eds.), *AIDS, Sexuality and Gender in Africa: Collective Strategies and Struggles in Tanzania and Zambia* (pp. 1-24). London: Routlegde.

Baylies, C., & Bujra , J. (Eds.). (2000). *AIDS, Sexuality and Gender in Africa: Collective Strategies and Struggles in Tanzania and Zambia*. London: Routlegde.

Becker, H. (2004). Efundula: Women's Initiation, Gender and Sexual Identities in Colonial and Post-Colonial Namibia. In S. Arnfred (Ed.), *Re-thinking Sexualities in Africa* (pp. 35-56). Uppsala: The Nordic African Institute.

Beechey, V., & Whitelegg, E. (1986). *Women in Britain Today*. Milton Keynes: Open University Press.

Bell, L. (1998). Public and Private Meanings in Diaries: Researching Family and Childcare. In J. Ribbens & R. Edwards (Eds.), *Feminist Dilemmas in Qualitative Research* (pp. 72-86). London: Sage.

Bennet, J. (Ed.). (2005). *Killing a Virus With a Stone? Research on the Implementation of Policies Against Sexual Harassment in Southern African Higher Education*. Cape Town: Africa Gender Institute, University of Cape Town.

BERA. (2004). *Revised Ethical Guidelines for Educational Research*. Southwell: British Educational Research Association.

Bergen, R. K. (1993). Interviewing Survivors of Marital Rape: Doing Feminist Research on Sensitive Topics. In C. M. Renzetti & R. M. Lee (Eds.), *Researching Sensitive Topics* (pp. 197-211). Newburry Park: Sage.

Birch, M., & Miller, T. (2000). Inviting Intimacy: The Interview as Therapeutic Opportunity. *International Journal of Social Research Methodology: Theory and Practice*, 3(3), 189-202.

Birch, M., & Miller, T. (2002). Encouraging Participation: Ethics and Responsibilities. In M. Mauthner & M. Birch, et al. (Eds.), *Ethics in Qualitative Research* (pp. 91-106). London: Sage.

Birch, M., Miller, T., Mauthner, M., & Jessop, J. (2002). Introduction. In M. Birch & T. Miller, et al. (Eds.), *Ethics in Qualitative Research* (pp. 1- 13). London: Sage.

Blackmore, J. (1999). *Troubling Women: Feminism, Leadership and Educational Change*. Buckingham: Open University Press.

Bollag, B. (2001, March 2). African Universities Begin to Face the Enormity of their Losses to AIDS. *The Chronicle of Higher Education*, pp. a45-a47.

Bond, S. (2000). Culture and Feminine Leadership. In M. L. Kearney (Ed.), *Women, Power and the Academy: From Rhetoric to Reality* (pp. 79-85). Paris: UNESCO.

Boyd, E. R. (2002). 'Being There': Mothers Who Stay at Home, Gender and Time. *Women's Studies International Forum*, 25(4), 463-470.

Brannen, J. (1988). The Study of Sensitive Subjects. *Sociological Review*, 36, 552-563.

Brannen, J., Meszaros, G., Moss, P., & Poland, G. (1994). *Employment and Family Life: A Review of Research in the UK* (1980-1994). London: Institute of Education - University of London.

Brooks, A., & Mackinnon, A. (Eds.). (2001). *Gender and the Restructured University*. Buckingham: Open University Press.

Brown, A., & Dowling, P. (1998). *Doing Research/Reading Research: A Mode of Interrogation for Education*. London: The Falmer Press.

Browne, K. (2005). Snowball Sampling: Using Social Networks to Research Non-Heterosexual Women. *International Journal of Social Research Methodology: Theory and Practice*, 8(1), 47-60.

Bujra , J., & Baylies, C. (2000). Responses to the AIDS Epidemic in Tanzania and Zambia. In C. Baylies & J. Bujra (Eds.), *AIDS, Sexuality and Gender in Africa* (pp. 25-59). London: Routlegde.

Bujra, J., & Baylies, C. (1995). Discourses of Power and Empowerment in the Fight Against HIV/AIDS in Africa. In P. Aggleton & P. Davies, et al. (Eds.), *AIDS: Safety, Sexuality and Risk*. London: Taylor and Francis.

Burgess, R. G. (1982). The Unstructured Interview as a Conversation. In R. G. Burgess (Ed.), *Field Research: A Sourcebook and Field Manual*. London: Unwin Hyman.

Burgess, R. G. (1988). Conversations with a Purpose: The Ethnographic Interview in Educational Research. In R. G. Burgess (Ed.), *Studies in Qualitative Methodology* (Vol. 1, pp. 137-156). London: Jai Press.

Burke, P. J. (2002). *Accessing Education: Effectively Widening Participation*. Staffordshire: Trentham Books.

Campbell, C. (2003). *Letting Them Die: Why HIV/AIDS Prevention Programmes Fail*. Cape Town: The International African Institute.

Campbell, C., Nair, Y., & Maimane, S. (2006). AIDS Stigma, Sexual Moralities and The Policing of Women and Youth in South Africa. *Feminist Review*, 83, 132-138.

Caplan, P. (1993). Introduction to the Volume. In D. Bell & P. Caplan, et al. (Eds.), *Gendered Fields* (pp. 19-27). London and New York: Routlegde.

Chapman, V. L. (2003). On 'Knowing One's Self' Self-Writing, Power and Ethical Practice: Reflections From an Adult Educator. *Studies in the Education of Adults*, 35(1), 35-53.

Chatzifotiou, S. (2000). Conducting Qualitative Research on Wife Abuse: Dealing with the Issue of Anxiety. *Sociological Research Online*, 5(2), 9.4 paragraphs.

CHE, & UNESCO. (2004, November 22 to 24). Developing Policies and Practices for Mainstreaming HIV and AIDS in Institutions of Higher Education, Kenya Institute of Education, Nairobi.

Cheemeh, P. E., Montoya, I. D., Essien, J. E., & Ogungbade, G. O. (2006). HIV/AIDS in The Middle East: A Guide To a Proactive Response. *The Journal of the Royal Society for the Promotion of Health*, 126(4), 165-171.

Chege, F. (2004, 2nd February). *Teachers' Gendered Lives, HIV/AIDS and Pedagogy*. Paper presented at the Beyond Access: Pedagogic Strategies for Gender Equality and Quality Basic Education in Schools, Nairobi.

Chetty, D. (2000). *Institutionalising the Response to HIV/AIDS in South African University Sector: A SAUVCA Analysis*. Pretoria: South African Universities Vice - Chancellors Association (SAUVCA).

Chilisa, B., Bennell, P., & Hyde, K. (2001). *The Impact of HIV/AIDS on the University of Botswana: Developing a Comprehensive Strategic Approach*. Retrieved 30th October, 2003, from the World Wide Web: http://www.ub.bw/initiatives/hivawareness/Truth/ImpactofHIVAIDS.pdf

CIA. (2012)."The World Factbook-Kenya", available at: https://www.cia.gov/library/publications/the-world-factbook/geos/ke.html. Accessed on 31 July 2012.

Ciambrone, D. (2003). *Women's Experiences with HIV/AIDS: Mending Fractured Selves*. New York: The Haworth Press.

Clandinin, J., & Connelly, F. M. (1998). Personal Experience Methods. In N. K. Denzin & Y. S. Lincoln (Eds.), *Collecting and Interpreting Qualititative Materials* (pp. 150-178). London: Sage.

Clinton, H. R. (2003). Living History. London: Headline.

Coate, K. (1999). Feminist Knowledge and the Ivory Tower: A Case Study. *Gender and Education*, 11(2), 141 - 159.

Cockburn, C. (2002). Resisting Equal Opportunities: The Issues of Maternity. In S. Jackson & S. Scott (Eds.), *Gender: A Sociological Reader* (pp. 180-191). London: Routledge.

Coleman, M. (2002). *Women as Head Teachers: Striking a Balance.* Stoke on Trent: Trentham books.

Columbia University Press. 2000. *The Columbia Encyclopedia, 6th edition.* Boston, MA: Houghton Mifflin.

Commonwealth Secretariat. (2002). *Gender Mainstreaming in HIV / AIDS: Taking a Multisectoral Approach.* London: Commonwealth Secretariat.

Cook, J., & Fonow, M. (1990). Knowledge and Women's Interests: Issues of Epistemology and Methodology in Feminist Sociological Research. In J. Nielsen (Ed.), *Feminist Research Methods* (pp. 70-93). Boulder: West View Press.

Corden, A., Sainsbury, R., Sloper, P., & Ward, B. (2005). Using a Model of Group Psychotherapy to Support Research on Sensitive Topics. *International Journal of Social Research Methodology: Theory and Practice,* 8(2), 151-160.

Cosslett, T., Lurry, C., & Summerfield, P. (2000). Introduction. In T. Cosslett & C. Lurry, et al. (Eds.), *Feminism and Autobiography: Texts, Theories, Methods* (pp. 1-21). London: Routlegde.

Crosby, C. (1992). Dealing with Differences. In J. Butler & J. W. Scott (Eds.), *Feminist Theorize the Political* (pp. 130-143). New York: Routlegde.

Currie, J., Thiele, B., & Harris, P. (2002). *Gendered Universities in Globalised Economies: Power, Career and Sacrifice.* Lexington Books.

Daily Nation. (2004, February 12). AIDS: Employers Must Act. *Daily Nation,* p. 8.

Davies, B. (1993). *Shards of Glass: Children Reading and Writing Beyond Gender Identities.* Sydney: Allen and Unwin.

Davies, C. (1996). The Sociology of Professions and the Profession of Gender. *Sociology,* 30(4), 661-678.

Deem, R. (2003). Gender, Organizational Cultures and the Practices of Manager-Academics in UK Universities. *Gender Work and Organization*, 10(2), 239-259.

Delphy, C., & Leonard, D. (1992). *Familiar Exploitation: A New Analysis of Marriage in Contemporary Western Societies*. Cambridge: Polity Press.

Delphy, C., & Leonard, D. (2002). The Variety of Work Done by Wives. In S. Jackson & S. Scott (Eds.), *Gender: A Sociological Reader* (pp. 170-179). London: Routledge.

Doucet, A., & Mauthner, N. (2002). Knowing Responsibly: Linking Ethics, Research, Practice and Epistemology. In M. Mauthner & M. Birch, et al. (Eds.), *Ethics in Qualitative Research* (pp. 123-145). London: Sage Publications.

Du Bois, B. (1983). Passionate Scholarship: Notes on Values Knowing and Methods in Feminist Social Science. In G. Bowles & K. R. Duelli (Eds.), *Theories of Women's Studies* (pp. 105-116). London: Routlegde and Kegan Paul.

Dube, M. W. (2004). HIV / AIDS and Other Challenges to Theological Education in the New Millennium. In G. LeMarquand & J. Galgalo (Eds.), *Theological Education in Contemporary Africa* (pp. 105-130). Eldoret: Zapf Chancery.

Duncombe, J., & Jessop, J. (2002). 'Doing Rapport' and the Ethics of 'Faking Friendship'. In M. Mauthner & M. Birch, et al. (Eds.), *Ethics in Qualitative Research* (pp. 107-122). London: Sage.

Dunn, L. (1991). Research Alert! Qualitative Research May Be Hazardous to Your Health. *Qualitative Health Research*, 1, 388-392.

Duongsaa, U. (2004, June). *Development, Gender, HIV/AIDS and Adult Education: Linkages, Lessons Learnt, and Challenges*. Paper presented at the Gender, Education and Development: Beyond Access Seminar, University of East Anglia, Norwich, UK.

Edwards, R., & Ribbens, J. (1998). Living on the Edges: Public Knowledge, Private Lives, Personal Experiences. In R. Edwards & J. Ribbens (Eds.), *Feminist Dilemmas in Qualitative Research: Public Knowledge and Private Lives* (pp. 1-23). London: Sage.

Elkins, C. (2005). *Imperial Reckoning: The Untold Story of Britain's Gulag in Kenya.* New York: Henry Holt and Company, LLC.

Esu-Williams, E. (1995). Individual and Collective Responsibility. In B. Schenider & N. Stoller (Eds.), *Women Resisting AIDS: Feminist Strategies for Empowerment.* Philadelphia: Temple University Press.

Finch, J., & Mason, J. (1993). *Negotiating Family Responsibilities.* London: Tavistock.

Fogelberg, P., Hearn, J., Husu, L., & Mankkinen, T. (1999). Hard Work in The Academy: Introduction. In P. Fogelberg & J. Hearn, et al. (Eds.), *Hard Work in the Academy: Research and Interventions on Gender Inequalities in Higher Education* (pp. 11-19). Helsinki: Helsinki University Press.

Foucault, M. (1978). *The History of Sexuality: An Introduction* (R. Hurley, Trans. Vol. 1). London: Penguin Books Ltd.

Francis, D., & Francis, E. (2006). Raising Awareness of HIV-Related Stigma and Its Associated Prejudice and Contradiction. *South African Journal for Higher Education,* 20(1), 44-55.

Garland, D. (2001, September). *Challenges to Capacity Building in Africa: Health and Gender Issues.* Paper presented at the Developing Global Capacity Through International Education, Sydney.

GHC. (2005). *Faith in Action: Examining the Role of Faith Based Organisations in Addressing HIV/AIDS.* Washington DC: Catholic Medical Mission Board.

Gichure, P., I. (2006). AIDS Stories As a Process of Healing. In A. Chepkwony, K (Ed.), *Religion and Health in Africa: Reflections for Theology in the 21st Century* (pp. 99-104). Nairobi: Paulines Publications, Africa.

Gillham, B. (2000a). *Case Study Research Methods*. London: Continuum.

Gillham, B. (2000b). *The Research Interview*. London: Continuum.

Gold, A. (1995). Working with Silences: Planning Management Development Programs Which Work For Women Too. In K. Hamalainen & D. Oldroyd, et al. (Eds.), *Making School Improvement Happen* (pp. 99-113). Helsinki: University of Helsinki.

Gold, A. (2001). The Philosophical Framework : Women Into Educational Management. In D. Elsner & A. Gold, et al. (Eds.), *International Program for Women into Educational Management: Training of Trainer Material and Workshop Strategies* (pp. 15-26). Heinola: Department of Education and Science, Ireland.

Gold, A., Unterhalter, E., & Morley, L. (2002). Managing Gendered Change in Commonwealth Universities. Vistas: *Journal of Humanities and Social Sciences*, 1(1), 55-71.

Goldberger, N. R., Clinchy, B. M., Belenky, M. F., & Tarule, J. M. (1987). Women's Ways of Knowing: On Gaining a Voice. In P. Shaver & C. Hendridk (Eds.), *Sex and Gender* (pp. 201-228). Newbury Park: Sage Publications.

Greed, C. (1990). The Professional and The Personal: A Study of Women Quantity Surveyors. In L. Stanley (Ed.), *Feminist Praxis* (pp. 145-155). London: Routlegde.

Green, G. (1996). Stigma and Social Relationships of People with HIV: Does Gender Make a Difference? In L. Sherr & C. Hankins, et al. (Eds.), *AIDS as a Gender Issue: Psychosocial Perspectives* (pp. 46-63). Oxon: Taylor and Francis.

Griffiths, M. (1998). *Educational Research for Social Justice: Getting off the Fence*. Buckingham: Open University Press.

Grunberg, L. (2001). *Good Practice in Promoting Gender Equality in Higher Education in Central and Eastern Europe*. Bucharest: UNESCO.

Gupta, G. R., Whelan, D., & Allendorf, K. (2003). *Integrating Gender into HIV and AIDS Programmes* (Vol. 2004). Washington DC: WHO.

Hall, V. (1996). *Dancing On The Ceiling: A Study of Women Managers In Education*. London: Paul Chapman Publishing.

Harding, S. (1987). *Introduction: Is There a Feminist Method? In S. Harding (Ed.), Feminism and Methodology* (pp. 1-14). Milton Keynes: Open University Press.

Harding, S. (1991). *Whose Science? Whose Knowledge? Thinking From Women's Lives*. Milton Keynes: Open University Press.

Hatt, S. (1999b). Establishing a Research Career. In S. Hatt & J. Kent, et al. (Eds.), *Women, Research and Careers* (pp. 111-133). Houndmills: Macmillan Press Ltd.

Hatt, S., Kent, J., & Britton, C. (1999). *Women, Research and Careers*. Houndmills: Macmillan Press Ltd.

Hays, S.-J., & Murphy, G. (2003). Gaining Ethical Approval for Research into Sensitive Topics: 'Two Strikes and You're Out?' *British Journal of Learning Disabilities*, 31, 181-189.

Henry, K. (1996, May). Women and AIDS Care: Coping with "Triple Jeopardy". *AIDS Captions, Family Health International*, Volume 3.

Hochschild, A. (2002). Emotional Labour. In S. Jackson & S. Scott (Eds.), *Gender: A Sociological Reader* (pp. 193-196). London: Routledge.

Hoehler-Fatton, C. (1996). *Women of Fire and Spirit : History, Faith and Gender in Roho Religion In Western Kenya*. Oxford: Oxford University Press.

Hollway, W., & Jefferson, T. (2000). *Doing Qualitative Research Differently: Free Association and Interview Method*. London: Sage.

Holmes, M. (2000). When Is The Personal Political? The President's Penis and Other Stories. *Sociology*, 34(2), 305-321.

Holstein, J. A., & Gubrium, J. F. (1995). *The Active Interview*. Thousand Oaks: Sage.

hooks, b. (1994). *Teaching to Transgress: Education as the Practice of Freedom*. New York: Routledge.

hooks, b. (2000). *Feminist Theory: From Margin to Center* (Second ed.). London: Pluto Press.

House-Midamba, B. (1990). *Class Development and Gender Inequality in Kenya, 1963-1990* (Vol. 20). New York: The Edwin Mellen Press.

Hubbard, G., Backet-Milburn, K., & Kemmer, D. (2001). Working with Emotion: Issues For The Researcher in Fieldwork and Teamwork. *International Journal of Social Research Methodology: Theory and Practice*, 4(2), 119-137.

Hughes, B., McKie, L., Hopkins, D., & Watson, N. (2005). Love's Labours Lost? Feminists, The Disabled People's Movement and An Ethic of Care. *Sociology*, 39(2), 258-273.

Hughes, C. (2002). *Key Concepts in Feminist Theory and Research*. London: Sage.

Humpreys, M., & Gutenby, B. (1999). Exploring Gender, Management Education and Careers: Speaking in the Silences. *Gender and Education*, 11(number 3), 281 - 294.

Hunter, S. (2003). *Who Cares? AIDS in Africa*. Houndmills: Palgrave.

Jones, C., & Rupp, S. (2000). Understanding The Carers' World: A Biographical Interpretive Case Study. In P. Chamberlayne & J. Bornat, et al. (Eds.), *The Turn to Biographical Methods in Social Science: Comparative Issues and Examples* (pp. 276-289). London: Routlegde.

Kaleeba, N., & Ray, S. (1997). *We Miss You All*. Harare: Women and AIDS Support Network.

Kamaara, E. K. (2005). *Youth Sexuality and HIV/AIDS: A Kenyan Experience.* Eldoret: AMECEA Publications.

Kamau, N. (2001). *The Status of Women and Management in Kenyan Universities: A Study of One Private University.* Unpublished MA Dissertation, University of London, Institute of Education, London.

Kamau, N. (2002). The Status of Women in Higher Education Management: A Study of One Private University in Kenya. *Eastern Africa Journal of Humanities and Sciences,* 2.(1).

Kamau, N. (2003). Do Women Bring a Different Perspective Into Political Leadership? In M. Nzomo (Ed.), *Perspectives on Gender Discourse: Women in Politics, Challenges of Democratic Transition in Kenya* (pp. 103-118). Nairobi: Heinrich Boll Foundation.

Kamau, N. (2004a). Making Women and Girls More Visible in the Fight Against HIV/AIDS in Kenya. In P. Achola, P.W. & J. Shiundu, O., et al. (Eds.), *Governance, Society and Development in Kenya* (pp. 135-157). Eldoret: Moi University Press and OSSREA.

Kamau, N. (2004b, 5th May). *The Use of Transformative Interventions in Reducing Gender Based Vulnerability to HIV and AIDS in Kenya: a Kenyan Woman's Perspective.* Paper presented at the HIV/ AIDS, Politics, Prevention, Treatment and Care, Good Enough College, London.

Kamau, N. (2006). Invisibility, Silence and Absence: A Study of The Account Taken by Two Kenyan Universities of The Effects of HIV and AIDS on Senior Women Staff. *Women Studies International Forum,* 29, 612-619.

Kamau, N. (2010). *Women and Political Leadership in Kenya: Ten Case Studies.* Nairobi. Heinrich Boll Foundation

Kanake, L. (1995). *Gender Disparities Among Academic Staff in Kenyan Public Universities.* Nairobi: Education Research Series.

KANCO. (2000). *Information Package on Gender and HIV/AIDS.* Nairobi: Kenya AIDS NGOs Consortium supported by USAID through FHI.

Kanogo, T. (2005). *African Womanhood in Colonial Kenya: 1900-50.* Nairobi: EAEP.

Kanter, R. M. (1977). *Men and Women of the Corporation.* New York: Basic Books.

Kearney, M.-L. (2000). Overview: From Rhetoric to Reality. In M.-L. Kearney (Ed.), *Women, Power and the Academy: From Rhetoric to Reality* (pp. 1-17). Paris: UNESCO.

Kelly, B. (2003). *HIV/AIDS a Response of Love: Words of Encouragement and Hope.* Nairobi: Paulines Publications Africa.

Kelly, L., Burton, S., & Regan, L. (1994). Researching Women's Lives or Studying Women's Oppression? Reflections on What Constitutes Women's Research. In M. Maynard & J. Purvis (Eds.), *Researching Women's Lives From a Feminist Perspective* (pp. 27-48). Portsmouth: Taylor and Francis.

Kelly, M. J. (2001, March). *Challenging The Challenger: Understanding and Expanding the Response of Universities in Africa to HIV/AIDS. ADEA Working Group on Higher Education.* Retrieved 15th November, 2003, from the World Wide Web: http://www.adeanet.org/publications/wghe/Univ_Aids_Rept_en.html

Kelly, M. J. (2003a, September). *The HIV/AIDS Context for the Leadership Response.* Paper presented at the HIV/AIDS: Government Leaders in Namibia Responding to the HIV/AIDS Epidemic, Safari Court Hotel, Windhoek, Namibia.

Kelly, M. J. (2003b). The Significance of HIV/AIDS for Universities in Africa. *Journal of Higher Education in Africa,* 1(1), 1-36.

Kelly, M. J. (2004a, 22nd - 24th November). *Theory and Practice of Mainstreaming HIV/AIDS in Institutions of Higher Learning.* Paper presented at the Developing Policies and Practices for Mainstreaming HIV and AIDS in Institutions of Higher Learning, KIE, Nairobi.

Kelly, M. J. (2004b, 22nd -24th November). *Why Institutions of Higher Learning Must Respond to HIV/AIDS*. Paper presented at the Developing Policies and Practices for Mainstreaming HIV and AIDS in Institutions of Higher Learning, KIE, Nairobi.

Kenway, J., Willis, S., Blackmore, J., & Rennie, L. (1994). Making 'Hope Practical' Rather Than 'Despair Convincing': Feminist Post-Structuralism, Gender Reform and Educational Change. *British Journal of Sociology of Education*, 15(2), 187-210.

Kenyatta, J. (1938). *Facing Mount Kenya: The Tribal Life of the Gikuyu*. London: Secker and War burg.

Khamisi, W. (2005, 22nd to 26th August). *The Staff Gender Status at Moi University - Kenya*. Paper presented at the Women and Management in Higher Education Training of Trainers Workshop, Imperial Botanical Hotel Entebbe Uganda.

Khasiani, A. S. (2000). Women in Academia. In J. Oshumuwe (Ed.), *Women and Leadership in Kenya* (pp. 9-23). Nairobi: Konrad -Adenauer-Foundation.

Khathide, A. G. (2003). Teaching and Talking About Sexuality: A Means of Combating HIV/AIDS. In M. W. Dube (Ed.), *HIV/AIDS and the Curriculum: Methods of Integrating HIV/AIDS in the Theological Programmes* (pp. 3-9). Geneva: WCC.

Kiiti, N. (1993, December). Swimming Against the Current: Maintaining a Balance Between Building a Successful Career and Making Home is a Stressful Exercise. *Lady*, 17-18.

Kiluva-Ndunda, M. M. (2001). *Women's Agency and Educational Policy: The Experiences of The Women of Kilome, Kenya*. New York: State University of New York Press.

Kjeldal, S.-E.-R., Jennifer - Sheridan, Alison. (2005). Deal-Making and Rule-Breaking: Behind the Façade of Equity in Academia. *Gender and Education*, 17(4), 431-448.

KNBS. (2010). *Kenya: 2009 Population and Housing Census Highlights*. Nairobi: KNBSenya National Bureau of Statistics.

Knight, P. T. (2002). *Small-Scale Research*. London: Sage.

Kolawole, M. M. E. (1997). *Womanism and African Conciousness*. Trento: Africa World Press Inc.

Kuria, M. (Ed.). (2003). *Talking Gender: Conversations With Kenyan Women Writers*. Nairobi: PJ.

Kvale, S. (1996). *Interviews: An Introduction to Qualitative Research Interviewing*. London: Sage.

Kwesiga, C. J. (2002). *Women's Access to Higher Education in Africa: Uganda's Experience*. Kampala: Fountain Publishers.

Lee, R. M., & Renzetti, C. M. (1993). The Problems of Researching Sensitive Topics: An Overview and Introduction. In C. M. Renzetti & R. M. Lee (Eds.), *Researching Sensitive Topics* (pp. 3-13). Newburry Park: Sage.

Lee, S. S. (2001). "A Root Out of a Dry Ground": Resolving the Researcher/Researched Dilemma. In J. Zeni (Ed.), *Ethical Issues in Practitioner Research* (pp. 61-71). New York: Teachers College Press.

Leonard, D. (2001). *A Woman's Guide to Doctoral Studies*. Buckingham: Open University Press.

Leonard, D., & Speakman, M. A. (1986). Women in the Family: Companions or Caretakers. In V. Beechey & E. Whitelegg (Eds.), *Women in Britain Today* (pp. 8-76). London: Open University Press.

Lewis, M. G. (1993). *Without a Word: Teaching Beyond Women's Silence*. New York: Routledge.

Lewis, S. (2003, 3rd January). *Text of UN briefing by Stephen Lewis on HIV/AIDS in Africa*. Retrieved 4th February, 2004, from the World Wide Web: http://www.worldrevolution.org/article/279

Lindow, M. (2006, September 1). In Zambia, Treating The Sympton of Silence: A University Fights Not Only AIDS, But the Stigma of the Disease. *Chronicle of Higher Education*, A68-A71.

Lipinge, S., Hofnie, K., & Friedman, S. (2004). *The Relationship Between Gender Roles and HIV Infection in Namibia*. Windhoek: University of Namibia Press.

Lorber, J. (2000). Guarding the Gates: The Micropolitics of Gender. In M. Kimmel, S. & A. Aronson (Eds.), *The Gendered Society Reader* (pp. 270 - 294). New York: Oxford University Press.

Lovett, M. (1989). Gender Relations, Class Formation and the Colonial State in Africa. In J. L. Parpart & K. A. Staudt (Eds.), *Women and The State in Africa* (pp. 22-46). Boulder: Lynne Rienner Publishers.

Luke, C. (1994). Women in The Academy: The Politics of Speech and Silence. *British Journal of Sociology of Education*, 15(2), 211-230.

Lund, H. (1998). *A Single Sex Profession: Female Staff Numbers in Commonwealth Universities*. London: CHEMS.

Maathai, M. W. (2006). *Unbowed: A Memoir*. London: William Heinemann.

Mabokela, R. O. (2003). 'Donkeys of the University': Organizational Culture and Its Impact on South African Women Administrators. *Higher Education*, 46(Number: 2), 129 -145.

Machera, M. (2004). Opening a Can of Worms: A Debate on Female Sexuality in The Lecture Theatre. In S. Arnfred (Ed.), *Re-Thinking Sexualities in Africa* (pp. 157-170). Uppsala: The Nordic Africa Institute.

Mackinnon, C. (1997). Feminism, Marxism, Method, and the State: An Agenda for Theory. In D. Meyers (Ed.), *Feminist Social Thought: A Reader* (pp. 64-91). New York: Routledge.

Magambo, J. K. (2000). *HIV/AIDS in Jomo Kenyatta University of Agriculture and Technology: A Case Study*. Nairobi: ADEA, Higher Education Working Group, World Bank.

Manchester, J. (2001, 4-6 April). *The HIV Epidemic in South Africa: Personal Views of Positive People.* Paper presented at the Politics of Gender and Education, Institute of Education, University of London.

Manya, M. (2000). *Equal Opportunities Policy (Gender): A Means to Increasing the Number of Female Senior Managers and Decision Makers at the University of Nairobi.* Unpublished MA Dissertation, University of London, Institute of Education, London.

Marcus, R. (1993). *Gender and HIV and AIDS in Sub-Saharan Africa: The Cases of Uganda and Malawi* (number 13). Brighton: Centre for Development Studies, University College, Swansea.

Marshall, A. (1994). Sensuous Sapphires: A Study of The Social Construction of Black Female Sexuality. In M. Maynard & J. Purvis (Eds.), *Researching Women's Lives From a Feminist Perspective* (pp. 106-124). Portsmouth: Taylor and Francis.

Mason, J. (2002). *Qualitative Researching* (second ed.). London: Sage.

Mauthner, M. (1998). Bringing Silent Voices into a Public Discourse: Researching Accounts of Sister Relationships. In J. Ribbens & R. Edwards (Eds.), *Feminist Dilemmas in Qualitative Research: Public Knowledge and Private Lives* (pp. 39-57). London: Sage.

Mauthner, M. (2000). Snippets and Silences: Ethics and Reflexivity in Narratives of Sistering. *Social Research Methodology*, 3(4), 287-306.

Mauthner, M., Birch, M., Jessop, J., & Miller, T. (Eds.). (2002). *Ethics in Qualitative Research.* London: Sage.

Mauthner, N., & Doucet, A. (1998). Reflections on a Voice-Centered Relational Method: Analysing Maternal and Domestic Voices. In J. Ribbens & R. Edwards (Eds.), *Feminist Dilemmas in Qualitative Research: Public Knowledge and Private Lives* (pp. 119-146). London: Sage.

Mavin, S., & Bryans, P. (2002). Academic Women in the UK: Mainstreaming our Experiences and Networking for Action. *Gender and Education*, 14(3), 235-250.

Maynard, M. (1993). Feminism and The Possibilities of a Postmodern Research Practice. *British Journal of Sociology of Education*, 14(3), 327-331.

Maynard, M. (1994). Methods, Practice and Epistemology: The Debate About Feminism and Research. In M. Maynard & J. Purvis (Eds.), *Researching Women's Lives From a Feminist Perspective*. London: Taylor and Francis.

Maynard, M. (1995). Beyond The 'Big Three': The Development of Feminist Theory Into The 1990s. *Women's History Review*, 4(3), 259-281.

Maynard, M., & Purvis, J. (1994b). Doing Feminist Research: Introduction. In M. Maynard & J. Purvis (Eds.), *Researching Women's Lives from a Feminist Perspective* (pp. 1-9). London: Taylor and Francis.

Mbilinyi, M., & Kaihula, N. (2000). Sinners and Outsiders: The Drama of AIDS in Rungwe. In C. Baylies & J. Bujra (Eds.), *AIDS, Sexuality and Gender in Africa: Collective Strategies and Struggles in Tanzania and Zambia* (pp. 77-95). London: Routlegde.

Mbiti, J. S. (1975). *Introduction to African Religion*. London: Heinneman.

McFadden, P. (2003). Sexual Pleasure as Feminist Choice. *Feminist Africa: Changing Cultures* (2), 50 - 60.

McKie, L., Bowlby, S., & Gregory, S. (2001). Gender, Caring and Employment in Britain. *Journal of Social Policy*, 30(2), 233-258.

McKie, L., Bowlby, S., & Gregory, S. (2004). Starting Well: Gender and Health in the Family Context. *Sociology*, 38(3), 593-611.

Merrill, B. (1999). *Gender, Change and Identity: Mature Women Students in Universities*. Aldershot: Ashgate.

Miller, T. (1998). Shifting Layers of Professional, Lay and Personal Narratives: Longitudinal Childbirth Research. In J. Ribbens & R. Edwards (Eds.), *Feminist Dilemmas in Qualitative Research: Public Knowledge and Private Lives* (pp. 58-71). London: Sage.

Miller, T., & Bell, L. (2002). Consenting to What? Issues of Access, Gate-Keeping and Informed Consent. In M. Mauthner & M. Birch, et al. (Eds.), *Ethics in Qualitative Research* (pp. 53-69). London: Sage Publications Ltd.

Miroiu, M. (2003). *Guidelines for Promoting Gender Equity in Higher Education in Central and Eastern Europe.* Bucharest: UNESCO.

Moore, D. (1999). Thresholds, Hurdles and Ceilings: Career Patterns of Women in Israeri Academia. In P. Fogelberg & J. Hearn, et al. (Eds.), *Hard Work in the Academy* (pp. 116-123). Helsinki: Helsinki University Press.

Morley, L. (1999). *Organising Feminisms: The Micro Politics of The Academy.* Houndmills: Macmillan Press.

Morley, L. (2000). *The Micropolitics of Gender in the Learning Society. Higher Education in Europe,* Volume: 25 (Number: 2), 229 - 235.

Morley, L. (2003a). *Quality and Power in Higher Education.* Berkshire: SRHE and Open University Press.

Morley, L. (2003b). *Sounds, Silences and Contradictions: Gender Equity in Commonwealth Higher Education.* London: Institute of Education.

Morley, L., & Walsh, V. (Eds.). (1996). *Breaking Boundaries: Women in Higher Education* (first ed.). London: Taylor & Francis.

Morley, L., Gunawardena, C., Kwesiga, C. J., Lihamba, A., Odejide, A., Shackelton, L., & Sorhaindo, A. (2005). *Gender Equity in Commonwealth Higher Education: An Examination of Sustainable Interventions in Selected Commonwealth Universities.* London: Institute of Education and DfID.

Moyles, J. (2002). Observation as a Research Tool. In M. Coleman & A. R. J. Briggs (Eds.), *Research Methods in Educational Leadership and Management* (pp. 172-195). London: Paul Chapman.

Mufune, P. (2003). Changing Patterns of Sexuality in Northern Namibia: Implications for Transmission of HIV/AIDS. *Culture Health and Sexuality: An international Journal for Research, Intervention and Care*, 5(5), 425-438.

Mullens, A. (2003, October). AIDS at African Universities. *UNI - World - International Affairs Magazine of the Association of Universities and Colleges of Canada* (AUCC), 1 and 3.

Mutiswa, S. (2006, February 3). I Lost My Wife to Another Woman. *Saturday Nation*, pp. 12-13.

NACC. (2003). *Mainstreaming Gender into the Kenya National HIV/ AIDS Strategic Plan 2000-2005* (Policy document). Nairobi: National AIDS Control Council.

NACC and NASCOP. (2012). *Kenya AIDS Epidemic update 2011.* Nairobi: National AIDS Control Council.

Ndirangu, M. (2006, 26th April). An Act Most Cruel. *Daily Nation.*

Nelson, N. (1987). 'Selling Her Kiosk': Kikuyu Notions of Sexuality and Sex for Sale in Mathare Valley, Kenya. In P. Caplan (Ed.), *The Cultural Construction of Sexuality* (pp. 217-239). London: Tavistock Publications.

Nias, J., Southworth, G., & Yeomans, R. (1989). *Staff Relationships in the Primary School.* London: Cassell Educational Limited.

Nyanchwo, F. (2005, 22nd -26th August). *Gender Situation in Makerere University.* Paper presented at the Women and Management in Higher Education Training of Trainers Workshop, Imperial Botanical Hotel Entebbe Uganda.

Nyutho, E., Mubuu, K., & Mbindyo, J. (2005). *HIV/AIDS in Kenyan Universities: A Comparative Study on HIV/AIDS Interventions in Kenyan Universities* (Draft report). Nairobi: Links CBO.

Nzioka, C. (2000). *The Impact of HIV/AIDS on the University of Nairobi*. Nairobi: ADEA.

Nzomo, M. (2003a). Introduction. In M. Nzomo (Ed.), *Perspectives on Gender Discourses* (pp. 9-16). Nairobi: Heinrich Boll Foundation.

Nzomo, M. (2003b). Taking Stock: Women's Performance in Kenya's Parliamentary Politics in the 2002 General Elections. In M. Nzomo (Ed.), *Perspectives on Gender Discourses* (pp. 17-32). Nairobi: Heinrich Boll Foundation.

Oakley, A. (1990). Interviewing Women: A Contradiction in Terms. In H. Roberts (Ed.), *Doing Feminist Research*. London: Routlegde.

Oakley, A. (1992). *Social Support and Motherhood*. Oxford: Blackwell.

Oakley, A. (2001). Foreword. In A. Brooks & A. Mackinnon (Eds.), *Gender and the Restructured University* (pp. xi - xiv). Buckingham: Open University Press.

Oakley, A. (2002). *Gender On Planet Earth* (first ed.). Cambridge: Polity Press.

Obbo, C. (1980). *African Women: Their Struggle for Economic Independence*. London: Zedd Press.

Ochola-Ayayo, A. (1997). HIV/AIDS Risk Factors and Changing Sexual Practices in Kenya. In T. S. Weisner & Bradley Candice, et al. (Eds.), *African Families and the Crisis of Social Change* (pp. 109 - 124). Westport: Bergin and Garvey.

Odhiambo, R. (2005, 22nd to 26th August 2005). *Institutional Report on Status of Women in The University: A Case of Egerton University, Kenya*. Paper presented at the Women and Management in Higher Education Training of Trainers Workshop, Imperial Botanical Hotel Entebbe Uganda.

Odinga, O. (1967). *Not Yet Uhuru: An Autobiography.* London: Heinemann.

Oduol, W., & Kabira, W. M. (2000). The Mother of Warriors and Her Daughters: The Women's Movement in Kenya. In B. G. Smith (Ed.), *Global Feminisms Since 1945* (pp. 101-118). London: Routledge.

Okello, R. (2003). *Why Leadership is Key in Ending Violence Against Women.* AWCFS. Retrieved 26th October, 2005, from the World Wide Web: http://www.awcfs.org/contentcreation/noviolence/noviolence1.html

Olenja, J. M. (1999). Assessing Community Attitude Towards Home Based Care for People with AIDS (PWAS) in Kenya. *Journal of Community Health,* 24(3), 187-199.

Onsongo, J. K. (2000). *'Publish or Perish': An Investigation Into Academic Women's Access to Research and Publication in Kenyan Universities.* Unpublished MA Dissertation, University of London, Institute of Education, London.

Onsongo, J. K. (2005). *"Outsiders Within": Women's Participation in University Management in Kenya.* Unpublished PhD, University College London, London.

Opie, A. (1992). Qualitative Research, Appropriation of the 'Other' and Empowerment. *Feminist Review* (40), 55-69.

O'Sullivan, S. (1996). *I Used to be Nice: Sexual Affairs.* New York: Cassell.

Otaala, B. (2000). *HIV/AIDS: The Challenge for Tertiary Institutions in Namibia,* Proceedings of a Workshop held from October 9th to 11th 2000, at Safari Hotel Court Conference Centre. Windhoek.

Ouston, J. (1993). *Women in Education Management.* London: Longman.

Outshoorn, J. (2002). Gendering The "Greying" of Society: A Discourse Analysis of The Care Gap. *Public Administration Review,* 62(2), 185-196.

Owino, P. O. (2004). *Study of African Universities' Responses to HIV/AIDS: The Case of Kenya.* Nairobi: Association for the Development of Education in Africa.

Parker, R., & Aggleton , P. (2003). HIV and AIDS Related Stigma and Discrimination: A Conceptual Framework and Implications for Action. *Social Science and Medicine,* 57, 13-24.

Parr, J. (1998). Theoretical Voices and Women's Own Voices: The Stories of Mature Women Students. In J. Ribbens & R. Edwards (Eds.), *Feminist Dilemmas in Qualitative Research: Public Knowledge and Private Lives* (pp. 87-102). London: Sage Publications.

Pereira, C. (2003). "Where Angles Fear to Tread" Some Thoughts on Patricia McFadden's "Sexual Pleasure as Feminist Choice". *Feminist Africa: Changing Cultures* (2), 61-65.

Phaswana-Mafuya, M. N. (2005). HIV/AIDS Situational Analysis Among Tertiary Institutions in the Eastern Cape. *South African Journal for Higher Education,* 19(6).

Phaswana-Mafuya, M. N., & Peltzer, K. (2006). Percieved HIV/AIDS Impact Among Higher Education Institutions in the Eastern Cape. *South African Journal for Higher Education,* 20(1), 143-156.

Phoenix, A. (1994). Practising Feminist Research: The Intersection Between Gender and 'Race' in the Research Process. In M. Maynard & J. Purvis (Eds.), *Researching Women's Lives From a Feminist Perspective* (pp. 49-71). London: Taylor and Francis.

Piot, P. (2005). *Speech of the UNAIDS Executive Director. UNAIDS.* Retrieved 14th June, 2005, from the World Wide Web: Http:wwww.UNAIDS.ORG

Preece, J., & Ntseane, G. (2004). Using Adult Education Principles for HIV/AIDS Awareness Intervention Strategies in Botswana. *International Journal of Lifelong Education,* 23(1), 5-22.

Probert, B. (2005). 'I Just Couldn't Fit It In': Gender and Unequal Outcomes in Academic Careers. *Gender, Work and Organizations,* 12(1), 50-72.

PWC. (2004). *HIV/AIDS: What is Business Doing?* Nairobi: PWC.

Ramazanoglu, C., & Holland, J. (2002). *Feminist Methodology.* London: Sage Publications.

Rankka, K. (1998). *Women and the Value of Suffering: An Aw(e)ful Rowing Toward God.* Minnesota: Liturgical Press.

Reinharz, S. (1992). *Feminist Methods in Social Research.* Oxford: Oxford University Press.

Reiss, M. J. (2000). *Understanding Science Lessons: Five Years of Science Teaching.* Buckingham: Open University Press.

Reskin, B. F. (2000). Bringing The Men Back In: Sex Differentiation and The Differentiation of Women's Work. In M. Kimmel, S. & A. Aronson (Eds.), *The Gendered Society Reader* (pp. 257- 270). New YorK: Oxford University Press.

Reynolds, T. (2002). On Relations Between Black Female Researchers and Participants. In T. May (Ed.), *Qualitative Research in Action* (pp. 300-309). London: Sage.

Ribbens, J. (1998). Hearing My Feeling Voice: An Autobiographical Discussion of Motherhood. In J. Ribbens & R. Edwards (Eds.), *Feminist Dilemmas in Qualitative Research: Public Knowledge and Private Lives* (pp. 24-38). London: Sage Publications.

Robson, C. (2002). *Real World Research* (2nd ed.). Oxford: Blackwell Publishing.

Romanin, S., & Over, R. (1993). Australian Academics: Career Patterns, Work Roles and Family Life Cycle Commitments of Men and Women. *Higher Education*, 26(4), 411 - 429.

Rossouw, H. (2005, February 11). University of Zambia Offers Free Anti-AIDS Drugs to Students, Staff and Faculty Members. *The Chronicle of Higher Education*, A40.

Roth, N. L., & Hogan, K. (Eds.). (1998). *Gendered Epidemic: Representations of Women in The Age of AIDS.* New York: Routlegde.

Rotham, B. K. (1986). Reflections on Hard Work. *Qualitative Sociology*, 9, 48-53.

Ruijs, A. (1993). *Women Managers in Education: A Worldwide Report.* Bristol: The Staff College, Coombe Logde Reports.

Sabatier, R. (1988). *Blaming Others.* London: Panos Publications Ltd.

Sarpong, P. K. (2005). The Cultural Practices Influencing The Spread of HIV/AIDS. In M. Czerny (Ed.), *AIDS and The African Church* (pp. 43-48). Nairobi: Paulines Publications Africa.

Scott, J. W. (1988). Deconstructing Equality-versus-Difference: Or The Uses of Poststruturalist Theory for Feminism. *Feminist Studies*, 14(1), 33-50.

Scott, J. W. (1990). Deconstructing Equality-versus Difference. In M. Hirsch & E. F. Keller (Eds.), *Conflicts in Feminism* (pp. 134-148). New York: Routledge.

Shahidian, H. (2001). "To be Recorded in History": Researching Iranian Underground Political Activists in Exile. *Qualitative Sociology*, 24(1), 55-81.

Shelp, E. E., & Sunderland, R. H. (1987). *AIDS and the Church.* Philadelphia: Westminster Press.

Sherr, L., Hankins, C., & Bennet, L. (Eds.). (1996). *AIDS as a Gender Issue.* London: Taylor and Francis.

Shisanya, C. R. A. (2002). The Impact of HIV/AIDS on Women in Kenya. In M. Getui & M. M. Theuri (Eds.), *Quest for Abundant Life in Africa* (pp. 45-75). Nairobi: Acton Publishers.

Singh, J. S. (2002). *Women and Management in Higher Education: A Good Practice Handbook.* Paris: UNESCO.

Singh, J. S. (2003). *Still a Single Sex Profession?* London: Association of Commonwealth Universities.

Siplon, P. (2005). AIDS and Patriarchy: Ideological Obstacles to Effective Policy Making. In A. S. Patterson (Ed.), *The African State and The AIDS Crisis* (pp. 17 - 36). Burlington: Ashgate.

Skeggs, B. (1994). Situating The Production of Feminist Ethnography. In M. Maynard & J. Purvis (Eds.), *Researching Women's Lives from a Feminist Perspective* (pp. 72-92). London: Taylor and Francis.

Skeggs, B. (1995). Theorising, Ethics and Representation in Feminist Ethnography. In B. Skeggs (Ed.), *Feminist Cultural Theory* (pp. 190-206). Manchester: Manchester University Press.

Skeggs, B. (1997). *Formations of Class and Gender: Becoming Respectable*. London: Sage.

Smit, P. (2006). *Leadership in South African Higher Education: A Multifaceted Conceptualization*. Unpublished PhD, University of London: Institute of Education, London.

Smith, A., & McDonagh, E. (2003). *The Reality of HIV and AIDS*. Dublin: Trocaire, Veritas and Cafod.

Smith, D., E. (2002). Institutional Ethnography. In T. May (Ed.), *Qualitative Research in Action* (pp. 17-52). London: Sage.

St. Pierre, E. A. (2000). Post-structural Feminism in Education: An Overview. *Qualitative Studies in Education*, 13(5), 477-515.

Stamp, P. (1986). Kikuyu Women's Self -Help Groups: Towards an Understanding of Relations Between Sex-Gender Systems and Mode of Production in Africa. In C. Robertson & I. Berger (Eds.), *Women and Class in Africa* (pp. 22-47). New York: African Publishing Company.

Stamp, P. (1989). *Technology: Gender and Power in Africa*. Ottawa: ONT and IDRC.

Standing, K. (1998). Writing the Voices of the Less Powerful. In J. Ribbens & R. Edwards (Eds.), *Feminist Dilemmas in Qualitative Research: Public Knowledge and Private Lives* (pp. 186-202). London: Sage Publications.

Stanko, E. (1994). Dancing With Denial: Researching Women and Questioning Men. In M. Maynard & J. Purvis (Eds.), *Researching Women's Lives From a Feminist Perspective* (pp. 93-105). London: Taylor and Francis.

Stanley, L. (1991). Feminist Auto/Biography and Feminist Epistemology. In J. Aron & S. Walby (Eds.), *Out of the Margins: Women's Studies in The 1990s* (pp. 204-219). London: Taylor and Francis.

Stanley, L. (Ed.). (1990). *Feminist Praxis: Research, Theory and Epistemology in Feminist Sociology.* London: Routledge and Kegan.

Stanley, L., & Wise, S. (1983). 'Back Into The Personal' : Our Attempt to Construct Feminist Research. In G. Bowles & R. Klein-Duelli (Eds.), *Theories of Women's Studies* (pp. 192-211). London: Routledge.

Stanley, L., & Wise, S. (1990). Method, Methodology and Epistemology in Feminist Research Processes. In L. Stanley (Ed.), *Feminist Praxis: Research, Theory and Epistemology in Feminist Sociology* (pp. 20 - 60). London: Routledge.

Stanley, L., & Wise, S. (1993). *Breaking Out Again.* London: Routlegde.

Steedman, C. (1986). *Landscape For a Good Woman: A Story of Two Lives.* London: Virago.

Tamale, S. (2005). Eroticism, Sensuality and "Women's Secrets" Among the Baganda: A Critical Analysis. *Feminist Africa* (5), 5-36.

Tang, N. (2002). Interviewer and Interviewee Relationship. *Sociology,* 36(3), 703-721.

Teferra, D., & Altbach, P., G. (2004). African Higher Education: Challenges for the 21st Century. *Higher Education,* 47, 21-50.

Thapar-Bjorkert, S., & Henry, M. (2004). Reassessing the Research Relationship: Location, Position and Power in Field-work Accounts. *International Journal of Social Research Methodology: Theory and Practice*, 7(5), 363-381.

The Columbia Electronic Encyclopaedia. (2005). *Kenya. Columbia University Press.* Retrieved 27th October, 2005, from the World Wide Web: http://www.infoplease.com/ce6/world/A0859116.html?mail-10-27

Thiam, A. (1986). *Speak Out, Black Sisters! Black Women and Oppression in Black Africa* (D. S. Blair, Trans.). London: Pluto Press.

Thomas, C. (1993). Deconstructing The Concept of Care. *Sociology*, 27(4), 649-669.

Travers, M., & Bennet, L. (1996). AIDS, Women and Power. In L. Sherr & C. Hankins, et al. (Eds.), *AIDS as a Gender Issue: Psychosocial Perspectives* (pp. 64- 77). Oxon: Taylor and Francis.

Treichler, P., & Warren, C. (1998). May Be Next Year: Feminist Silence and The AIDS Epidemic. In N. L. Roth & K. Hogan (Eds.), *Gendered Epidemic: Representations of Women in the Age of AIDS* (pp. 109-152). New York: Routlegde.

Udoto, P. (2004, 31st March). Access to AIDS Drugs in Doubt. *Daily Nation*, pp. 11.

Ulin, P., R., Robinson, E., T., Tolley, E. E., & McNeill, E. T. (2002). *Qualitative Methods: A field Guide for Applied Research in Sexual and Reproductive Health.* North Carolina: Family Health International.

UNAIDS. (2004a). *Global Estimates of HIV and AIDS As of End 2003. UNAIDS.* Retrieved 14th June 2005, from the World Wide Web: http:www.UNAIDS.org/bangkok2004/GAR2004_pdf/global

UNAIDS. (2004b). *Report on The Global AIDS Epidemic: Executive Summary.* Geneva: UNAIDS.

UNAIDS. (2005). *AIDS Epidemic Update. UNAIDS*. Retrieved 28th November, 2005, from www.UNAIDS.org.

UNAIDS. (2010a). *Global Report: UNAIDS Report on the Global AIDS Epidemic 2010*. Geneva: UNAIDS. Also available at http://www.unaids.org

UNAIDS. (2010b). *HIV and AIDS Estimates, 2009*. Available at http://www.unaids.org/en/regionscountries/countries/kenya. Accessed on 04 September 2012.

UNAIDS. (2011). *World AIDS Day Report 2011*. Geneva: UNAIDS.

Vliet, V. (1996). *The Politics of AIDS*. London: Bowerdean Publishing Company Ltd.

VSO. (2003). *Gendering AIDS: Women, Men, Empowerment, Mobilization. VSO*. Retrieved 20th January 2004, 2003, from the World Wide Web: http://www.vso.org.uk/advocacy/hivaids_gender.htm

Waller, M.-K. (2004). *The Silenced Realities of HIV/AIDS: Women's Experiences Through Changing Gender, Kinship and Moral Landscapes in Urban Zambia*. Unpublished PHD, School of Oriental and African Studies, London.

Warren, T. (2003). Class and Gender-Based Working Time: Time Poverty and The Domestic Division of Labour. *Sociology*, 37(4), 733-752.

WCC. (1997). *Facing AIDS: The Challenge, The Churches' Response*. Geneva: WCC.

Weiner, G. (1994). *Feminisms in Education: An Introduction*. Buckingham: Open University Press.

Wengraf, T. (2001). *Qualitative Research Interviewing: Biographic Narrative and Semi-Structured Methods*. London: Sage.

Wickham-Searl, P. (1992). Careers in Caring: Mothers of Children with Disabilities. *Disability, Handicap and Society*, 7(1), 5-16.

Williams, A. (1990). Reading Feminisms in Field Notes. In L. Stanley (Ed.), *Feminist Praxis* (pp. 253-261). London: Routlegde.

Wisker, G. (1996). *Empowering Women in Higher Education Management*. London: Kogan Page.

Wood, K. (2002). *An Ethnography of Sexual Health and Violence Among Township Youth in South Africa*. Unpublished PhD, London School of Hygiene and Tropical Medicine, London.

World Bank. (1989). *The Role of Women in Economic Development: Kenya*. Washington D.C: World bank.

World Bank. (2003). *The Kenya Strategic Country Gender Assessment*. Washington D.C: World Bank.

Wragg, T. (2002). Interviewing. In M. Coleman & A. R. J. Briggs (Eds.), *Research Methods in Educational Leadership and Management* (pp. 143-158). London: Paul Chapman.

Wyn, J., Acker, S., & Richards, E. (2000). Making a Difference: Women in Management in Australian and Canadian Faculties of Education. *Gender and Education, 12*(5), 435 - 447.

Yin, R. K. (2003). *Case Study Research: Design and Methods* (3rd ed.). London: Sage Publications.

Index

Zapf Chancery Tertiary Level Publications

A Guide to Academic Writing by **C. B. Peter** *(1994)*

Africa in the 21st Century by **Eric M. Aseka** *(1996)*

Women in Development by **Egara Kabaji** *(1997)*

Introducing Social Science: A Guidebook by **J. H. van Doorne** *(2000)*

Elementary Statistics by **J. H. van Doorne** *(2001)*

Iteso Survival Rites on the Birth of Twins by **Festus B. Omusolo** *(2001)*

The Church in the New Millennium: Three Studies in the Acts of the Apostles by **John Stott** *(2002)*

Introduction to Philosophy in an African Perspective by **Cletus N.Chukwu** *(2002)*

Participatory Monitoring and Evaluation by **Francis W. Mulwa and Simon N. Nguluu** (2003)

Applied Ethics and HIV/AIDS in Africa by **Cletus N. Chukwu** *(2003)*

For God and Humanity: 100 Years of St. Paul's United Theological College **edited by Emily Onyango** *(2003)*

Establishing and Managing School Libraries and Resource Centres by **Margaret Makenzi and Raymond Ongus** *(2003)*

Introduction to the Study of Religion by **Nehemiah Nyaundi** *(2003)*

A Guest in God's World: Memories of Madagascar by **Patricia McGregor** *(2004)*

Introduction to Critical Thinking by **J. Kahiga Kiruki** *(2004)*

Theological Education in Contemporary Africa edited by **GrantLeMarquand and Joseph D. Galgalo** *(2004)*

Looking Religion in the Eye **edited by Kennedy Onkware** *(2004)*

Computer Programming: Theory and Practice by **Gerald Injendi** *(2005)*

Demystifying Participatory Development by **Francis W. Mulwa** *(2005)*

Music Education in Kenya: A Historical Perspective by **Hellen A. Odwar** *(2005)*

Into the Sunshine: Integrating HIV/AIDS into Ethics Curriculum **edited by Charles Klagba and C. B. Peter** *(2005)*

Integrating HIV/AIDS into Ethics Curriculum: Suggested Modules **edited by Charles Klagba** *(2005)*

Dying Voice (An Anthropological Novel) by **Andrew K. Tanui** *(2006)*

Participatory Learning and Action (PLA): A Guide to Best Practice by **Enoch Harun Opuka** *(2006)*

Science and Human Values: Essays in Science, Religion, and Modern Ethical Issues **edited by Nehemiah Nyaundi and Kennedy Onkware** *(2006)*

Understanding Adolescent Behaviour by **Daniel Kasomo** *(2006)*

Students' Handbook for Guidance and Counselling by **Daniel Kasomo** *(2007)*

BusinessOrganization and Management: Questions and Answers by **Musa O. Nyakora** *(2007)*

Auditing Priniples: A Stuents' Handbook by **Musa O. Nyakora** *(2007)*

The Concept of Botho and HIV/AIDS in Botswana edited by **Joseph B. R. Gaie and Sana K. MMolai** *(2007)*

Captive of Fate: A Novel by **Ketty Arucy** *(2007)*

A Guide to Ethics by **Joseph Njino** *(2008)*

Pastoral Theology: Rediscovering African Models and Methods by **Ndung'u John Brown Ikenye** *(2009)*

The Royal Son: Balancing Barthian and African Christologies by **Zablon Bundi Mutongu** *(2009)*

AIDS, Sexuality, and Gender: Experiencing of Women in Kenyan Universities by **Nyokabi Kamau** *(2009)*

Modern Facilitation and Training Methodology: A Guide to Best Practice in Africa by **Frederick Chelule** *(2009)*

How to Write a Winning Thesis by **Simon Kang'ethe et al** *(2009)*

Absolute Power and Other Stories by **Ambrose Rotich Keitany** *(2009)*

Y'sdom in Africa: A Personal Journey by **Stanley Kinyeki** *(2010)*

Abortion and Morality Debate in Africa: A Philosophical Enquiry by **George Kegode** *(2010)*

The Holy Spirit as Liberator: A Study of Luke 4: 14-30 by **Joseph Koech** *(2010)*

Biblical Studies, Theology, Religion and Philosophy: An Introduction for African Universities, **Gen. Ed. James N. Amanze** *(2010)*

Modeling for Servant-Leaders in Africa: Lessons from St. Paul by **Ndung'u John Brown Ikenye** *(2010)*

HIV & AIDS, Communication and Secondary Education in Kenya by **Ndeti Ndati** *(2011)*

Disability, Society and Theology: Voices from Africa by **Samuel Kabue et al** *(2011)*

If You Have No Voice Just Sing!: Narratives of Women's Lives and Theological Education at St. Paul's University by **Esther Mombo And Heleen Joziasse** *(2011)*

Mutira Mission: An African Church Comes of Age in Kirinyaga, Kenya (1912-2012) by **Julius Gathogo** *(2011)*

The Bible and African Culture: Mapping Transactional Inroads by **Humphrey Waweru** *(2011)*

Karl Jaspers' Philosophy of Existence: Insights for Out Time by **Cletus N. Chukwu** *(2011)*

Diet of Worms: Quality of Catering in Kenyan Prisons by **Jacqueline Cheptekkeny Korir** *(2011)*

Our Father! An Indian Christian Prays the Lord's Prayer by **C. B. Peter** *(2011)*

African Christianity: The Stranger Within by **Joseph D. Galgalo** *(2012)*

A Handbook of African Church History by **Medard Rugyendo** *(2012)*

Project Planning and Management: A Kenyan Experience by **Zablon Bundi Mutongu and Lily Njanja** *(2012)*

Reading and Comprehension in the African Context: A Cognitive Enquiry by **Agnes Wanja Kibui** *(2012)*

Researching AIDS, Sexuality, and Gender (2nd Revised Edition) by **Nyokabi Kamau** *(2012)*

♦ ♦ ♦ ♦ ♦ ♦ ♦ ♦ ♦ ♦ ♦ ♦ ♦ ♦

Worldwide Distributors of Zapf Chancery Publications

AFRICAN BOOKS COLLECTIVE
(www.aricanbookscollective.com)
P. O. Box 721
Oxford OX1 9EN, UK

Tel: +44 (0) 1865 58 9756
Fax: +44 (0) 1865 412 341
US Tel: +1 415 644 5108

Customer Services

Please email to: orders@africanbookscollective.com

Marketing and Production: Justin Cox
justin.cox@africanbookscollective.com

US Customer Assistance: Carolina Bruno
carolina.bruno@africanbookscollective.com

For order within Kenya please email to: info@zapfchancery.org